NCLEX-RN®
IN A FLASH

Ray A. Gapuz, RN, MAN
Founder and Chairman
R.A. Gapuz Review Center, Inc.
Manila, Philippines

JONES AND BARTLETT PUBLISHERS
Sudbury, Massachusetts
BOSTON   TORONTO   LONDON   SINGAPORE

World Headquarters
Jones and Bartlett Publishers
40 Tall Pine Drive
Sudbury, MA 01776
978-443-5000
info@jbpub.com
www.jbpub.com

Jones and Bartlett Publishers Canada
6339 Ormindale Way
Mississauga, Ontario L5V 1J2
Canada

Jones and Bartlett Publishers International
Barb House, Barb Mews
London W6 7PA
United Kingdom

Jones and Bartlett's books and products are available through most bookstores and online booksellers. To contact Jones and Bartlett Publishers directly, call 800-832-0034, fax 978-443-8000, or visit our website www.jbpub.com.

Substantial discounts on bulk quantities of Jones and Bartlett's publications are available to corporations, professional associations, and other qualified organizations. For details and specific discount information, contact the special sales department at Jones and Bartlett via the above contact information or send an email to specialsales@jbpub.com.

Production Credits
Publisher: Kevin Sullivan
Acquisitions Editor: Emily Ekle
Acquisitions Editor: Amy Sibley
Associate Editor: Patricia Donnelly
Editorial Assistant: Rachel Shuster
Supervising Production Editor: Carolyn F. Rogers
Associate Marketing Manager: Ilana Goddess
Manufacturing and Inventory Control Supervisor: Amy Bacus
Composition and Interior Design: Shawn Girsberger
Cover Design: Kristin E. Ohlin
Cover Image: © wheatley/ShutterStock, Inc.
Printing and Binding: Malloy, Inc.
Cover Printing: Malloy, Inc.

6048

Printed in the United States of America
12 11 10 09 08   10 9 8 7 6 5 4 3 2 1

AUTHOR'S NOTE

In my professional work as a lecturer and motivational speaker, I have been asked numerous questions. But questions from students regarding what to read in the weeks and days prior to the NCLEX® exam, are what I consider the most difficult to answer—or so I thought, until a 61-year-old post-craniotomy nurse approached me to ask for help so she could pass her nursing exam.

The main challenge for me was to come up with a review program that suited her age, attention span, and learning needs. This is how this book came to being. It contains the core concepts that I prepared to help the 61-year-old post-craniotomy nurse to realize her dream—to pass her exam. *NCLEX-RN® in a Flash* contains 311 functional concepts that are essential for the nurse to remember before taking the NCLEX-RN®.

Functional concepts are ideas that bridge the gap between the information contained in textbooks and the concepts covered in nursing exams. This book has been written to provide you with a comprehensive coverage of the concepts that are the subject matter of the NCLEX-RN®. The strength of this book is in its format, which enables you to recall theoretical concepts and relate these concepts to NCLEX-RN® questions in a short period of time, within 24 hours!

The first nurse to use this book read it exactly 24 hours before his scheduled test and he passed! What is amazing about his experience is that he was out of nursing for almost 15 years as he opted to work as an aerobics instructor. In his words, "the book lives up to its title: The 24-hour guide for passing the NCLEX-RN®."

This book has helped thousands of nurses in the Philippines, the Middle East, and some parts of Asia to pass the NCLEX-RN® and I'm certain it will also work for you!

Read on!

Ray A. Gapuz

iv

Subject

A subject line is found at the top of every page providing easy navigation throughout the book and a convenient snapshot into the topic area you are about to study.

Concept

The unique flowchart design begins with the presentation of a specific key concept within the subject area covered.

NCLEX-RN® Category

Found along the side of each page, the NCLEX-RN® category presents the specific exam blueprint area to which the question relates.

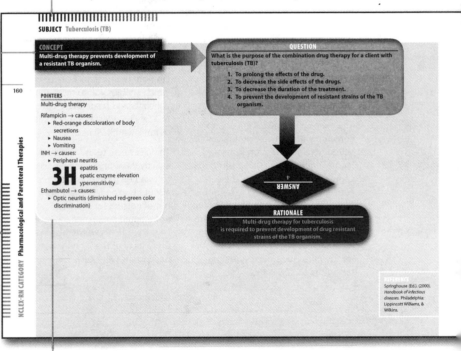

Pointers

An integral part of the learning process, "Pointers" reiterate the most important key messages, terms, and main ideas about the subject presented on each page.

Question and Answer

Like a flash card, thought-provoking questions appear on each page to provide insight into the questions that are found on the actual NCLEX-RN®. Test your knowledge in each unique subject area!

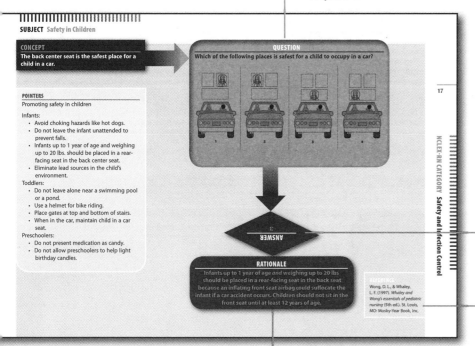

SUBJECT Safety in Children

CONCEPT
The back center seat is the safest place for a child in a car.

POINTERS
Promoting safety in children

Infants:
- Avoid choking hazards like hot dogs.
- Do not leave the infant unattended to prevent falls.
- Infants up to 1 year of age and weighing up to 20 lbs. should be placed in a rear-facing seat in the back center seat.
- Eliminate lead sources in the child's environment.

Toddlers:
- Do not leave alone near a swimming pool or a pond.
- Use a helmet for bike riding.
- Place gates at top and bottom of stairs.
- When in the car, maintain child in a car seat.

Preschoolers:
- Do not present medication as candy.
- Do not allow preschoolers to help light birthday candles.

QUESTION
Which of the following places is safest for a child to occupy in a car?

17

NCLEX-RN CATEGORY Safety and Infection Control

ANSWER
3

RATIONALE
Infants up to 1 year of age *and* weighing up to 20 lbs should be placed in a rear-facing seat in the back seat because an inflating front seat airbag could suffocate the infant if a car accident occurs. Children should not sit in the front seat until at least 12 years of age.

REFERENCE
Wong, D. L., & Whaley, L. F. (1997). *Whaley and Wong's essentials of pediatric nursing* (5th ed.). St. Louis, MO: Mosby-Year Book, Inc.

Answer

Once you have chosen your answer, compare it to the correct answer found upside down directly underneath the question.

Reference

References are included at the bottom of each page providing helpful information for test-takers looking for additional information on any subject found on the NCLEX-RN®!

Rationales

Rationales for each correct answer are presented to further promote understanding of the subject area.

CONCEPT

Clients with uncontrolled hemorrhage need to be treated immediately.

POINTERS

Conditions requiring immediate treatment

Cardiac arrest
Anaphylaxis
Multiple trauma
Profound shock

Poisoning
Active labor
Drug overdose
Severe head trauma, seizure
Severe respiratory distress

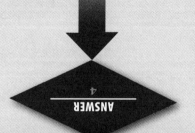

QUESTION

Which of the following conditions needs to be treated immediately?

1. Urinary retention.
2. Closed fracture.
3. Eye injury.
4. Continuous bleeding.

ANSWER

4

RATIONALE

A client with continuous bleeding may develop hypovolemic shock thereby needing immediate assessment and intervention.

REFERENCE

Grossman, V. G. A. (2003). *Quick Reference to Triage* (2nd ed.). Philadelphia: Lippincott Williams & Wilkins.

NCLEX-RN CATEGORY Management of Care

2

CONCEPT

Preventing the spread of infection is a consideration when delegating tasks to nurses.

POINTERS

Principles of delegation

5 Rights of Delegation*

- Right task to be delegated
- Under the right circumstances
- The right person to do the task
- The right direction and communication
- The right supervision to ensure that the task is carried out safely

*Source: National Council of State Boards of Nursing.

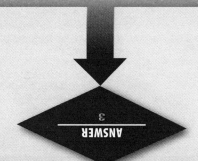

QUESTION

A staff nurse from the maternity ward is floated to the medical ward for the first four hours of the 3 to 11 pm shift. The charge nurse must assign three clients to the reassigned nurse. Which of the following clients is inappropriate to assign to this nurse?

1. A 12-year-old with rheumatic fever
2. A 6-year-old post cardiac catheterization
3. A 20-year-old with methicillin-resistant *Staphylococcus aureus*
4. A 15-year-old scheduled for an appendectomy

ANSWER

3

RATIONALE

A client with methicillin-resistant *Staphylococcus aureus* is considered infectious and therefore should not be delegated to the nurse. The nurse will be an agent in spreading the infection when the nurse returns to the maternity ward.

REFERENCE

Nettina, S. M. (2007). *The Lippincott manual of nursing practice* (8th ed., Philippine ed.). Philadelphia: Lippincott Williams & Wilkins.

CONCEPT

Ergonomics is the science of equipment design.

POINTERS

Principles of ergonomics

- Ergonomics is human-centered, transdisciplinary, and application-oriented.
- The aim of ergonomics is to achieve ease and efficiency at work.
- Gender, age, range of joint motions, strength, and grips of various population are essential factors to consider in designing products.

QUESTION

Which of the following outcome criteria indicates the effectiveness of the utilization of ergonomic principles in the workplace?

Select all that apply:

1. Reduced errors
2. Decreased feelings of fatigue
3. Decreased stress
4. Increased work productivity
5. Increased discomfort

ANSWER

1, 2, 3, 4

RATIONALE

Appropriately designed equipment reduces personnel errors; decreases fatigue, stress, and discomfort; and increases work productivity.

REFERENCE

SafeComputingTips. com. (2008). Homepage. Retrieved March 13, 2008, from http://www.safecomputingtips.com

1619
4369204

SUBJECT Diazepam (Valium)

CONCEPT

Valium is incompatible with any drug.

POINTERS

- Diazepam is an antianxiety agent; can be given as a muscle relaxant to clients in traction.
- Decreased anxiety and adequate sleep are indicators of effectiveness.
- Best taken before meals; food in the stomach delays absorption.
- Avoid driving or operating machinery; drug acts as central nervous system depressant.
- Avoid intake of alcohol and caffeine-containing foods; they alter the effect of the drug.
- Administer it separately; it is incompatible with any drug.
- Not given when a client is taking valerian or kava kava. Herbal sedatives potentiate the depressant effect of the drug.

QUESTION

Which of the following actions, if done by an RN, needs to be interrupted by the head nurse?

1. The RN administers Valium before meals
2. The RN raises the siderails of the client's bed after giving Valium
3. The RN mixes Valium and Demerol in one syringe
4. The RN instructs the client to avoid drinking coffee when taking Valium

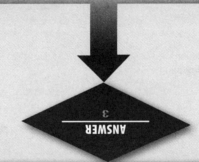

ANSWER 3

RATIONALE

Since Valium is incompatible with any drug, the RN should administer it using a separate syringe and avoid mixing it with other drugs.

REFERENCE

Karch, A. M. (2007). *2008 Lippincott's nursing drug guide.* Philadelphia: Lippincott Williams & Wilkins.

CONCEPT

Pain that is indicative of a complication is a nursing priority.

POINTERS

Some conditions manifested by pain are:

Ectopic pregnancy
- A sharp, dull, cramping, intermittent abdominal pain indicates rupture of the fallopian tubes.

Cholelithiasis
- Right upper-quadrant pain radiating to the shoulder blade

Renal calculi
- Pain from the costovertebral angle to the genitals

Abruptio placentae
- Painful dark red vaginal bleeding

QUESTION

Which of the following clients' complaint requires immediate nursing intervention?

1. A 40-year-old client with sharp, severe pain due to a renal stone, which is not relieved by analgesics
2. A 35-year-old client with fractured femur complaining of sharp chest pain
3. A 40-year-old client with cholelithiasis complaining of right-sided abdominal pain radiating to the shoulder blade
4. A client with ulcerative colitis having lower-left abdominal pain accompanied by bloody diarrhea

ANSWER

2

RATIONALE

Sharp chest pain in a client with a fractured femur is indicative of pulmonary embolism, which requires immediate nursing intervention.

REFERENCE

Nettina, S. M. (2007). *The Lippincott manual of nursing practice* (8th ed., Philippine ed.). Philadelphia: Lippincott Williams & Wilkins.

CONCEPT

The greatest single risk factor for the development of cancer is advancing age.

POINTERS

Risk factors for cancer

Carcinogens like asbestos, benzene, or radiation

Aging

Nutrition like high fat, low fiber, or salt cured food

Common viruses like:
- Human papilloma virus
  ‣ Cervical cancer
- Epstein-Barr virus
  ‣ Lymphoma
- Hepatitis B and C
  ‣ Liver cancer
- *Helicobacter pylori*
  ‣ Gastric cancer

Excessive alcohol intake combined with smoking

Race and gender

QUESTION

Which of the following clients is most at risk for cancer?

1. A 40-year-old African American female
2. A 20-year-old complaining of breast tenderness during menstruation
3. A 68-year-old Jewish male
4. A 36-year-old female who was hit in the chest with a ball 10 years ago

ANSWER

3

RATIONALE

A 68-year-old Jewish male is most at risk for cancer because aging is a significant factor.

REFERENCE

Nettina, S. M. (2007). *The Lippincott manual of nursing practice* (8th ed., Philippine ed.). Philadelphia: Lippincott Williams & Wilkins.

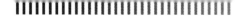

SUBJECT Saw Palmetto

CONCEPT

Saw palmetto is used as an oral treatment for benign prostatic hypertrophy.

POINTERS

Uses of saw palmetto

BPH
Asthma
Diuretic
Cough
Astringent
Bronchitis

Side effects
- Headache
- Diarrhea

QUESTION

Which of the following statements, if made by a client with benign prostatic hypertrophy, indicates the effectiveness of saw palmetto?

1. "It doesn't hurt me anymore when I urinate."
2. "I frequently urinate at night."
3. "My urinary stream has remained the same."
4. "I experience urinary dribbling occasionally."

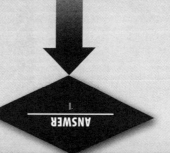

ANSWER

1

RATIONALE

Saw palmetto has an anti-spasmodic effect and is said to improve urine flow in clients with BPH.

7

NCLEX-RN CATEGORY **Basic Care and Comfort**

REFERENCE

Springhouse (Ed.). (2005). *Nursing herbal medicine handbook*. Philadelphia: Lippincott Williams & Wilkins.

SUBJECT Physical Assessment

NCLEX-RN CATEGORY   Management of Care

CONCEPT

The best place to auscultate for aortic patency is at the second intercostal space right sternal border.

POINTERS

Cardiac Sounds

S1—Created by the closure of the mitral and tricuspid valves

S2—Best heard at the apex of the heart (5th ICS)
- Created by the closing of the aortic and pulmonic valves
- Heard loudest at the base of the heart
- Aortic area is at the 2nd ICS right sternal border
- Pulmonic area is at the 2nd ICS left sternal border

S3—Gallop sound occurring during ventricular filling
- Normal in children and young adults
- May indicate heart failure in the elderly

S4—Gallop sounds heard during atrial contraction may indicate hypertrophy related to coronary artery disease, hypertension, or stenosis of the aortic valve

Opening snap—High pitched sound in the sternal border due to mitral stenosis

Ejection click—High pitched sound due to aortic stenosis

Murmurs—Sounds due to turbulent flow of blood that indicate congenital defect in the heart

Friction rubs—Harsh grating sounds related to pericarditis

QUESTION

Which area is appropriate for the nurse to auscultate to detect patency of the aorta?

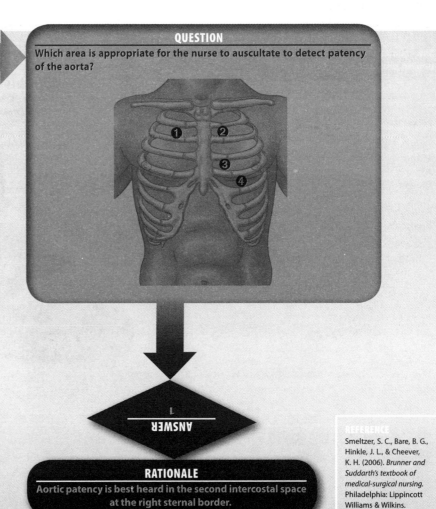

ANSWER

1

RATIONALE

Aortic patency is best heard in the second intercostal space at the right sternal border.

REFERENCE

Smeltzer, S. C., Bare, B. G., Hinkle, J. L., & Cheever, K. H. (2006). *Brunner and Suddarth's textbook of medical-surgical nursing.* Philadelphia: Lippincott Williams & Wilkins.

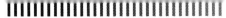

SUBJECT Triage

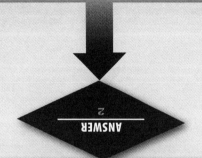

CONCEPT

Clients suffering from acute conditions should be assessed first.

POINTERS

Behavioral problems that require immediate interventions are as follows:

Aggression, inappropriate touching of others, indecent exposure

Setting fires, self-destruction, severe anxiety

Alcohol or drug use, attempts to leave the hospital

Physiologic alterations like failure to eat or sleep

QUESTION

Which of the following clients should the nurse assess first?

1. A client suffering from chronic schizophrenia who is withdrawn
2. A client with an acute attack of severe anxiety
3. A client with agoraphobia who stays in her room all day
4. A client with depression complaining of constipation

ANSWER

2

RATIONALE

A client with an acute anxiety attack is a threat to safety and should therefore be assessed first.

REFERENCE

Keltner, N. L., Bostrom, C. E., & Schweke, L. H. (2006). *Psychiatric nursing* (5th ed.). Philadelphia: Mosby.

SUBJECT Isolation Precautions

CONCEPT

A mask is used to limit the spread of infection for clients placed under airborne precautions.

POINTERS

Airborne precautions

Requirements:
- Private room
- Frequent handwashing
- Mask (particulate mask or N95 mask)

Indicated for:
- Measles
- Tuberculosis
- Varicella

If transport of the client is necessary, place a mask on the client, if possible.

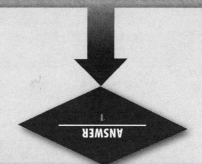

QUESTION

A registered nurse is assisting a client with measles for a chest x-ray. When transporting the client from the room to the x-ray department, the nurse should limit the spread of infection by performing which of the following interventions?

1. Placing a surgical mask on the client
2. Instructing all hospital personnel to wear a mask
3. Placing a particulate mask on the client
4. There are no special preparations needed for the client

ANSWER

1

RATIONALE

A client with measles requires airborne isolation precautions. The client should wear a surgical mask to prevent the spread of infection.

REFERENCE

Siegel, J. D., Rhinehart, E., Jackson, M., Chiarello, L., & the Healthcare Infection Control Practices Advisory Committee. (2007). *Guideline for isolation precautions.* Retrieved March 20, 2008 from www.cdc.gov/ncidod/ dhqp/pdf/guidelines/ Isolation2007.pdf

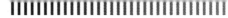
CONCEPT

Lyme disease is usually transmitted thru the bite of black legged ticks. The disease was initially diagnosed in Lyme, Connecticut.

POINTERS

- Lyme disease is a multi-system infectious syndrome commonly affecting the skin, nervous system, heart and joints.
- A bull's eye rash, usually found in moist parts of the body and described as "rounded rings" of rash, characterizes the disease.
- Ascertain if the client was exposed to deer ticks.
- Instruct the client to wear light colored clothing when going to the forest/woods or have himself/herself vaccinated.
- When bitten by a tick, remove it by exerting slow, steady pull upward and avoid squeezing it.

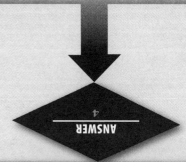

QUESTION

Who among the following clients is most at risk for Lyme disease?

1. A 15-year-old adolescent from New York
2. A 20-year-old pregnant client from California
3. A 40-year-old obese client from New Mexico
4. A 30-year-old male from Connecticut

ANSWER

4

RATIONALE

A person from Connecticut is at high risk for Lyme disease because the ticks causing the disease were initially found in that area.

11

NCLEX-RN CATEGORY **Physiological Adaptation**

REFERENCE

Nettina, S. M. (2007). *The Lippincott manual of nursing practice* (8th ed., Philippine ed.). Philadelphia: Lippincott Williams & Wilkins.

CONCEPT

Canned products contain high amounts of sodium.

POINTERS

Common sodium sources

- Spinach
- Shellfish
- Soup
- Seasonings
- Snack foods
- Salted products
- Smoked fish

QUESTION

Which of the following foods contains the highest amount of sodium?

1. Wheat bread
2. Instant oatmeal
3. Steamed corn
4. Fresh apples

ANSWER

2

RATIONALE

Convenience foods such as instant oatmeal and processed foods such as canned vegetables or meats are high in sodium content.

REFERENCE

Dudek, S. G. (2006). *Nutrition essentials for nursing practice* (5th ed.). Philadelphia: Lippincott Williams & Wilkins.

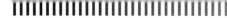

SUBJECT Tadalafil (Cialis)

CONCEPT
Cialis causes hypotension.

POINTERS
Common side effects of Cialis:

- Headache
- Upset stomach
- Backache
- Priapism

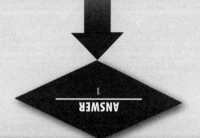

QUESTION
Which of the following should the nurse monitor in a client receiving tadalafil (Cialis)?

1. Blood pressure
2. Urine output
3. Urine specific gravity
4. Temperature

ANSWER
1

RATIONALE
When a client is receiving tadalafil (Cialis), the nurse should monitor the client's blood pressure carefully because the drug causes hypotension.

REFERENCE
Karch, A. M. (2007). *2008 Lippincott's nursing drug guide.* Philadelphia: Lippincott Williams & Wilkins.

NCLEX-RN CATEGORY **Pharmacological and Parenteral Therapies**

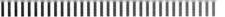
CONCEPT

A child discovers the hands at 3 months, has voluntary grasp at 6 months, develops the pincer grasp at 9 months, and has hand preference at 12 months.

POINTERS

1 month	The hands are kept in a fist
2–3 months	Discovers the hands, holds objects using the hands and brings them to the mouth
4 months	Grasps objects with both hands
6 months	Palmar grasp disappears
9 months	Uses index finger and thumb to hold objects
12 months	Hand dominance is apparent

QUESTION

Please arrange the following milestones of motor development in ascending order.

1. Prepares to use the right hand   _____
2. Plays with the fingers   _____
3. Picks up a Cheerio with the thumb and index finger   _____
4. Holds a toy with both hands   _____

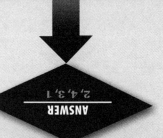

ANSWER

2, 4, 3, 1

RATIONALE

Growth and development are continuous processes and proceed in an orderly sequence. Development proceeds cephalocaudally, from proximal to distal parts and from gross to refined skills.

REFERENCE

Pillitteri, A. (2006). *Maternal and child health nursing* (5th ed.). Philadelphia: Lippincott Williams & Wilkins.

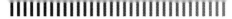
CONCEPT
Do not delegate any of the following tasks:

Assessment
Teaching
Evaluation

POINTERS
Principles of delegation

- RNs must not delegate a task that is within the scope of nursing practice.
- Assessment, discharge planning, or health education should not be delegated.

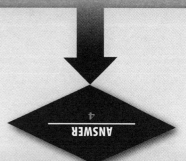

QUESTION
Which of the following interventions can be delegated to unlicensed assistive personnel by the registered nurse?

1. Assessing contractions in a client in labor
2. Evaluating the effects of antipsychotics in a client with schizophrenia
3. Teaching a diabetic client about foot care
4. Obtaining a routine urine specimen

ANSWER
4

RATIONALE
Obtaining a urine specimen is a routine standard procedure and therefore could be delegated. Anything that requires assessment, teaching, or evaluation should not be delegated.

REFERENCE
Steefel, L. (2007). Safety in numbers. *Nursing Spectrum, 17*(10), 40–41.

CONCEPT

An allergy to eggs or egg protein is a contraindication to influenza vaccine.

POINTERS

Age	Vaccine
• Birth–2 months	Hepatitis B 1
• 1–4 months	Hepatitis B 2
• 2 months	DTaP 1
	Hib1
	IPV 1
• 4 months	DTaP 2
	Hib 2
	IPV 2
• 6 months	DTaP 3
	Hib 3
• 6–18 months	Hepatitis B 3
	IPV or OPV 3
• 12–15 months	MMR
	Hib 3
	Var 1
• 15–18 months	DTaP 4
• 4–6 years	DTaP 5
	MMR 2
	IPV or OPV 4
• 11–12 years	Td 1

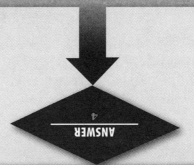

QUESTION

Before the administration of influenza vaccine, which of the following questions should the nurse ask the caregiver of the client?

1. "Is the child vomiting today?"
2. "Did you notice any strange behavior in the child lately?"
3. "Is the child able to drink from a glass?"
4. "Is the child allergic to eggs?"

ANSWER

4

RATIONALE

Before the administration of influenza vaccine, the nurse should ask the caregiver if the child has an allergy to eggs or chicken because the vaccine is inoculated from eggs.

REFERENCE
Karch, A. M. (2007). *2008 Lippincott's nursing drug guide*. Philadelphia: Lippincott Williams & Wilkins.

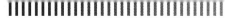

CONCEPT

The back center seat is the safest place for a child in a car.

POINTERS

Promoting safety in children

Infants:
- Avoid choking hazards like hot dogs.
- Do not leave the infant unattended to prevent falls.
- Infants up to 1 year of age and weighing up to 20 lbs. should be placed in a rear-facing seat in the back center seat.
- Eliminate lead sources in the child's environment.

Toddlers:
- Do not leave alone near a swimming pool or a pond.
- Use a helmet for bike riding.
- Place gates at top and bottom of stairs.
- When in the car, maintain child in a car seat.

Preschoolers:
- Do not present medication as candy.
- Do not allow preschoolers to help light birthday candles.

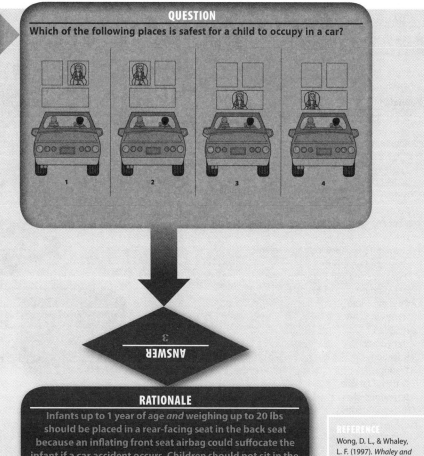

QUESTION

Which of the following places is safest for a child to occupy in a car?

1   2   3   4

ANSWER

3

RATIONALE

Infants up to 1 year of age *and* weighing up to 20 lbs should be placed in a rear-facing seat in the back seat because an inflating front seat airbag could suffocate the infant if a car accident occurs. Children should not sit in the front seat until at least 12 years of age.

REFERENCE

Wong, D. L., & Whaley, L. F. (1997). *Whaley and Wong's essentials of pediatric nursing* (5th ed.). St. Louis, MO: Mosby-Year Book, Inc.

17

NCLEX-RN CATEGORY **Safety and Infection Control**

CONCEPT

The clinical hallmark of sickle cell disease is acute pain due to vaso occlusive crisis.

QUESTION

Which of the following nursing diagnoses is the priority for a client with sickle cell disease?

1. Sensory–perceptual alteration
2. Pain
3. Fluid volume excess
4. Unilateral neglect

POINTERS

- Sickle cell anemia is a severe, chronic, hemolytic anemia inherited through the autosomal recessive pattern.
- Common manifestations:
  Jaundice
  Anemia
  Bone pain
  Signs of crisis
- Infarction (CVA) indicates vaso occlusive crisis
- Circulatory collapse indicates splenic sequestration crisis
- Decreased RBCs indicates aplastic crisis
- Precipitating factors of crisis:
  Cold exposure
  Hypoxia
  Acidosis
  Dehydration
  Infection
  Trauma
  Extreme fatigue
  Strenuous physical activities
- Nursing Priorities:
  - Pain relief
  - Promotion of hydration

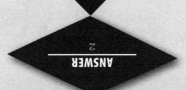

ANSWER

2

RATIONALE

Small blood vessels are occluded by the sickle-shaped cells causing distal ischemia and infarction, which results in severe bone pain and swollen joints. Hence, a priority nursing diagnosis is pain.

REFERENCE

Nettina, S. M. (2007). *The Lippincott manual of nursing practice* (8th ed., Philippine ed.). Philadelphia: Lippincott Williams & Wilkins.

SUBJECT Medication Administration

CONCEPT

When administering oral medications to young children, provide them a choice to give them a sense of control.

POINTERS

Key points to medication administration in children

- Do not pinch the child's nostrils when administering medication.
- Place the child in a sitting position with the head elevated when administering oral medication.
- Do not mix the medication with the entire amount of milk formula in a feeding bottle.
- Place a bandage over the puncture site when administering parenteral medications in toddlers and preschoolers to decrease the fear of body mutilation.

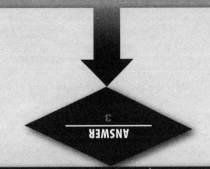

QUESTION

Which of the following approaches is the best way to administer oral medication to a toddler?

1. "Be a good boy, take this medicine now."
2. "If you don't take your medicine, you won't be able to go home."
3. "Would you like to take your medicine with milk or water?"
4. "Don't take your medicine, so you don't get well."

ANSWER

3

RATIONALE

Allowing the child to make a decision regarding his treatment is an appropriate approach because it gives the toddler a sense of autonomy.

REFERENCE

Wong, D. L., & Whaley, L. F. (1997). *Whaley and Wong's essentials of pediatric nursing* (5th ed.). St. Louis, MO: Mosby-Year Book, Inc.

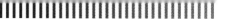

NCLEX-RN CATEGORY Pharmacological and Parenteral Therapies

CONCEPT

Some drugs are best absorbed when taken with the right drink.

POINTERS

- Iron → best taken with orange juice
- Fosamax → best taken with water
- Cyclosporine → avoid grapefruit juice
- Antidepressants → avoid acidic juices

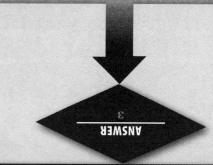

QUESTION

Which of the following clients needs further instruction from the nurse?

1. A client who is taking iron with orange juice
2. A client who is taking fosamax with mineral water
3. A client who is taking an antidepressant with orange juice
4. A client who is taking cyclosporine with water

ANSWER

3

RATIONALE

A client taking an antidepressant with orange juice needs further instruction because acidic juices decrease the absorption of antidepressants.

REFERENCE

Karch, A. M. (2007). *2008 Lippincott's nursing drug guide*. Philadelphia: Lippincott Williams & Wilkins.

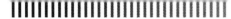
CONCEPT

Most neuroendocrine disorders require lifetime treatment with medications.

POINTERS

Conditions requiring lifetime medications

Anticholinesterase (Mestinon)	Myasthenia gravis
Antithyroid drugs (PTU)	Hyperthyroidism
Aspirin	Arthritis
AZT	AIDS
Dopaminergic agents (L-DOPA)	Parkinson's disease
Glucocorticoids (Deltasone)	Addison's disease
Glucocorticoid synthesis inhibitors (Mitotane)	Cushing's disease
Insulin (NPH, Regular)	Diabetes mellitus
Miotics (pilocarpine)	Glaucoma
Penicillin	Rheumatic heart disease
Thyroid supplement (Synthroid)	Hypothyroidism
Vitamin B$_{12}$	Pernicious anemia

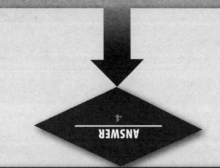

QUESTION

Which of the following statements, if made by a client with diabetes mellitus, reflects a need for further instructions?

1. "I will need some orange juice when I experience cold clammy skin."
2. "I will need to take my medication on time."
3. "I will need to take my medication for the rest of my life."
4. "I'm glad I will only take my medication until I reach 20."

ANSWER

4

RATIONALE

The client's statement "I'm glad I will only take my medication until I reach 20" indicates a need for further instruction because neuroendocrine disorders like diabetes mellitus require lifetime intake of medication.

REFERENCE

Karch, A. M. (2007). *2008 Lippincott's nursing drug guide*. Philadelphia: Lippincott Williams & Wilkins.

NCLEX-RN CATEGORY Pharmacological and Parenteral Therapies

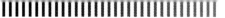

CONCEPT

In CPR, the shorter the time needed to deliver breaths, the faster the rescuer can resume chest compressions.

POINTERS

Basic life support for healthcare providers

1. Establish unresponsiveness
2. Open airway
   - Head tilt/chin lift (no injuries)
   - Jaw thrusts (neck injury is suspected)
3. Check for breathing; if not breathing, give two breaths
4. Check for pulse for no more than 10 seconds
   - Carotid (for child and adult)
   - Brachial or femoral (for infant)
5. If pulse is present but breathing is absent, provide rescue breathing:
   - 1 breath every 5 to 6 seconds → adult
   - 1 breath every 3 to 5 seconds → infant or child
6. If pulse is absent, begin chest compressions:
   - Compression–to–ventilation ratio 30:2 for all rescuers responding alone to victims of any age except newborns

Chest landmark:

Adult or child   - Lower part of the sternum; use both hands to compress

Infant   - Just below the nipple line; use two fingers to compress

QUESTION

Which of the following statements about cardiopulmonary resuscitation is not true?

1. Longer breaths are more effective in increasing oxygen levels in a client
2. Longer breaths delay performance of chest compression
3. Ideally, rescue breaths should be given in one second
4. It is better to deliver rescue breaths in a shorter time when performing CPR

ANSWER

1

RATIONALE

Longer breaths can delay the resumption of cardiac compression, thereby decreasing blood return to the heart.

REFERENCE

American Heart Association. (2005). Guidelines for cardiopulmonary resuscitation and emergency cardiovascular care. *Circulation*, 112(24, Suppl. 1), IV-12–IV-18, IV-154–IV-155.

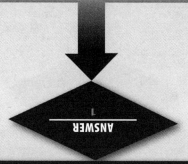

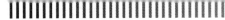

SUBJECT Chemotherapy

CONCEPT

Antiemetics are administered 30 minutes before chemotherapy.

POINTERS

Nursing care of clients undergoing chemotherapy

Check for any signs of infection and bleeding.

Hold antimetabolites like mercaptopurine (Purinethol), flouracil (5FU), floxuridine (FUDR), pentostatin (Nipent) if the WBC count is less than 4,000 cells/uL or if the platelet count is less than 75,000 u/L and refer to the physician because the drugs cause bone marrow depression.

Encourage client to increase oral fluid intake to 2 to 3 liters per day when on doxorubicin (Adriamycin), bleomycin (Blenoxane), dactinomycin (Cosmegen), cyclophosphamide (Cytoxan), and ifosfamide (Ifex) therapy to prevent hemorrhagic cystitis and severe renal impairment.

Monitor CBC, WBC, platelets, and uric acid levels.

Oral hygiene should be done with the use of a soft toothbrush to prevent gingival bleeding.

Temperature monitoring is done to detect early signs of infection.

Hold the use of aspirin, anticoagulants, and thrombolytic agents during the duration of chemotherapy to prevent bleeding.

Evaluate results of renal and liver function tests to assess for renal and hepatic impairment.

Reduce pain with IV administration as prescribed by diluting the medication or applying a warm compress on the injection site to distend the vein before giving the drug.

Administer antiemetic to prevent nausea and vomiting.

Perform pulmonary function tests.

You (the RN) should utilize standard precautions when caring for the client.

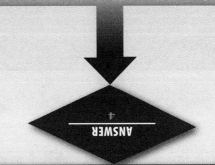

QUESTION

When is the best time to administer the antiemetic in a client undergoing chemotherapy?

1. When the client begins to feel nauseated
2. After completion of the treatment regimen
3. At the same time with the chemotherapeutic agent
4. Thirty minutes before chemotherapy is started

ANSWER
4

RATIONALE

To combat the most common side effect of chemotherapy, the nurse should administer the antiemetic approximately 30 minutes before the treatment is started.

REFERENCE

Karch, A. M. (2007). *2008 Lippincott's nursing drug guide*. Philadelphia: Lippincott Williams & Wilkins.

NCLEX-RN CATEGORY **Pharmacological and Parenteral Therapies**

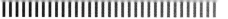

SUBJECT G6PD Deficiency

CONCEPT

G6PD deficiency is characterized by hemolysis.

POINTERS

- G6PD deficiency is an x-linked recessive condition characterized by hemolysis (destruction of RBCs).
- Jaundice is a common manifestation.
- Prepare the client for a blood transfusion.

QUESTION

G6PD deficiency can lead to which of the following conditions?

1. Leukopenia
2. Anemia
3. Bone marrow depression
4. Polycythemia

ANSWER

2

RATIONALE

G6PD is an x-linked recessive condition characterized by hemolysis that leads to anemia.

REFERENCE

Nettina, S. M. (2007). *The Lippincott manual of nursing practice* (8th ed., Philippine ed.). Philadelphia: Lippincott Williams & Wilkins.

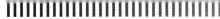

CONCEPT

Morphine sulfate causes more pain in clients with biliary conditions.

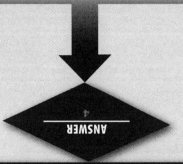

QUESTION

Which of the following conditions is not an indication for the use of morphine sulfate?

1. Heart failure
2. Myocardial infarction
3. Pulmonary edema
4. Pancreatitis

ANSWER

4

POINTERS

- Morphine is a narcotic agonist analgesic.
- Morphine is given to decrease anxiety in a client with pulmonary edema.
- It promotes venous pooling of blood in the periphery, so it decreases venous return to the heart.

RATIONALE

Morphine sulfate is absolutely contraindicated for a client with pancreatitis because it causes spasms of the Oddi's Sphincter, thereby increasing pain.

REFERENCE

Karch, A. M. (2007). *2008 Lippincott's nursing drug guide.* Philadelphia: Lippincott Williams & Wilkins.

NCLEX-RN CATEGORY **Pharmacological and Parenteral Therapies**

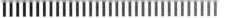
CONCEPT

Invasive diagnostic procedures require informed consent.

26

POINTERS

Procedures requiring informed consent:

- Surgical procedures
- Invasive procedures that involve entry into a body cavity
- Visualization or radiologic procedures with a contrast medium
- Procedures requiring the use of general anesthesia, local infiltration, and regional block

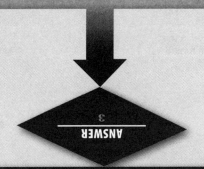

QUESTION

Which of the following procedures requires obtaining an informed consent?

1. KUB
2. EEG
3. Colonoscopy
4. Abdominal ultrasound

ANSWER

3

RATIONALE

Colonoscopy (the visualization of the entire large intestines, sigmoid colon, rectum, and anal canal) is an invasive procedure that requires an informed consent.

REFERENCE

Nettina, S. M. (2007). *The Lippincott manual of nursing practice* (8th ed., Philippine ed.). Philadelphia: Lippincott Williams & Wilkins.

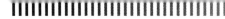

CONCEPT

In clients with feeding and drainage tubes, monitoring the intake and output is the priority.

POINTERS

- For clients with tube feedings, record the amount of formula actually taken by the client and report any decreased urine output.
- Maintaining the function of the tubes is a continuous responsibility of the nurse.

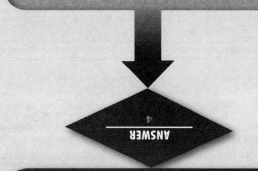

QUESTION

A client has an indwelling urinary catheter that drains an average of 40 ml of urine/hour. He also has a nasogastric tube in place and a chest tube attached to a 3-way bottle system. Which of the following actions is a nursing priority?

1. Assessing the patency of the chest tubes
2. Checking the placement of the nasogastric tube
3. Recording the amount of urine output
4. Monitoring the client's intake and output

ANSWER

4

RATIONALE

Monitoring the client's intake and output is a priority nursing action in a client with feeding and drainage tubes.

REFERENCE

Smeltzer, S. C., Bare, B. G., Hinkle, J. L., & Cheever, K. H. (2006). *Brunner and Suddarth's textbook of medical-surgical nursing*. Philadelphia: Lippincott Williams & Wilkins.

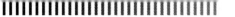

SUBJECT Thyroidectomy

CONCEPT

Hypocalcemia is manifested by a tingling sensation around the lips, Chvostek's sign, and Trousseau's sign.

POINTERS

Complications of thyroid surgery

4H emorrhage
ypothyroidism
ypoparathyroidism
ypocalcemia

- Assess for irritability, twitching, and spasms of hands and feet

QUESTION

Which of the following statements made by a client post-thyroidectomy indicates a complication?

1. "I have a tendency to limit my head movement."
2. "My facial muscles are relaxed."
3. "I have a tingling sensation around my lips."
4. "I feel some sense of pressure in my arm when the nurse takes my blood pressure."

ANSWER

3

RATIONALE

A tingling sensation around the lips is indicative of hypocalcemia due to accidental removal of the parathyroid glands during a thyroidectomy.

REFERENCE

Nettina, S. M. (2007). *The Lippincott manual of nursing practice* (8th ed., Philippine ed.). Philadelphia: Lippincott Williams & Wilkins.

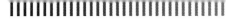
CONCEPT

Steroid therapy causes bone marrow depression.

POINTERS

Signs of infection like fever, redness, and swelling should be reported to the physician.

Trauma, a fall, or an automobile accident may precipitate adrenal failure, which can be managed by immediate injection of hydrocortisone (Solu-cortef).

Encourage good handwashing.

Restrict sodium intake and weigh the client daily.

Osteoporosis may result from long-term steroid therapy.

Instruct the client to avoid crowded areas and exposure to infection.

Diabetes mellitus, peptic ulcer, and viral infections are contraindications for steroid therapy.

QUESTION

A client with Addison's disease is having steroid therapy. The nurse knows that the client is at great risk for which of the following complications?

1. Fluid and electrolyte imbalance
2. Infection
3. Anorexia
4. Weight loss

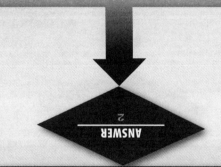

ANSWER

2

RATIONALE

Steroid therapy causes bone marrow depression, which leads to leukopenia (decreased white blood cells) increasing the client's risk for infection.

REFERENCE

Nettina, S. M. (2007). *The Lippincott manual of nursing practice* (8th ed., Philippine ed.). Philadelphia: Lippincott Williams & Wilkins.

29

NCLEX-RN CATEGORY **Pharmacological and Parenteral Therapies**

CONCEPT

In collecting a specimen for 24-hour collection, discard the first voided urine.

POINTERS

Steps in 24-hour urine collection

- Clean the perineal area before the client voids.
- Discard the first voided urine and note the time.
- Save the next voiding and all the client's urine in the next 24 hours.
- Save the last voiding and note the time.
- Refrigerate the urine specimen or keep it on ice.

QUESTION

The nurse is collecting a 24-hour urine specimen for Schilling's test. The first voiding is 50 ml. In the next 6 hours, the client's voided urine is 420 ml. The next 16 hours yielded an average of 60 ml. of urine per hour. The last voiding that occurred in the last 2 hours was 120 ml. How many ml of urine should the nurse document for the 24-hour urine collection?

1. 1,540 ml
2. 1,500 ml
3. 1,420 ml
4. 1,370 ml

ANSWER

2

RATIONALE

The computation is as follows:

420 ml – 2nd voiding
+ 960 ml – next 16 hrs.
+ 120 ml – last 2 hrs.
1500 ml – total amount of urine for 24-hour urine collection

The first voided urine of 50 ml should be discarded.

REFERENCE

Nettina, S. M. (2007). *The Lippincott manual of nursing practice* (8th ed., Philippine ed.). Philadelphia: Lippincott Williams & Wilkins.

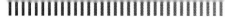

CONCEPT

Folic acid is found in green leafy vegetables.

POINTERS

Sources of folic acid

- Green leafy vegetables, dried peas and beans, seeds, liver, and orange juice
- The recommended dietary allowance for men and women is 400 ug/dL.
- The adult upper limit is 1,000 ug/dL.
- Deficiency may result in glossitis, diarrhea, macrocytic anemia, depression, confusion, fainting, and fatigue.

QUESTION

Which of the following food/s is/are good sources of folic acid?

Select all that apply:

1. Asparagus
2. Broccoli
3. Spinach
4. Strawberries
5. Tomatoes
6. Kiwi fruits
7. Peppers

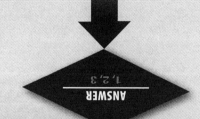

ANSWER

1, 2, 3

RATIONALE

Asparagus, broccoli, and spinach are vegetables that are rich in folic acid. Strawberries, tomatoes, kiwi fruits, and peppers are rich in vitamin C.

REFERENCE

Dudek, S. G. (2006). *Nutrition essentials for nursing practice* (5th ed.). Philadelphia: Lippincott Williams & Wilkins.

NCLEX-RN CATEGORY **Basic Care and Comfort**

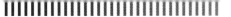
32

CONCEPT

Toddlers should be provided with toys that will encourage them to walk and talk.

POINTERS

- Toddlers usually engage in parallel play.
- They frequently change toys due to short attention span.
- Examples of toys for toddlers include push/ pull toys, blocks, toy telephone, trucks, and dolls.

Things to be avoided:

Pencil erasers, crayons, and play ponds. These may increase the incidence of aspiration and drowning.

QUESTION

Which of the following toys is most appropriate for a 15-month-old toddler?

1. Puzzles
2. Bicycle
3. Musical mobile
4. Push and pull toy car

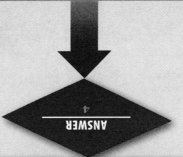

ANSWER

4

RATIONALE

The toys toddlers enjoy most are those they can play with by themselves and that require action, such as trucks they can make go, ducks they can pull, and toy telephones on which they can talk. These are all toys toddlers can control. Giving them a sense of power in manipulation is an expression of autonomy.

REFERENCE

Pillitteri, A. (2006). *Maternal and child health nursing* (5th ed.). Philadelphia: Lippincott Williams & Wilkins.

SUBJECT Iron Deficiency Anemia (IDA)

CONCEPT
Milk is a poor source of iron.

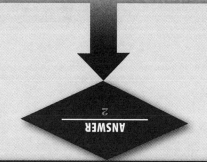

QUESTION
Which of the following statements, if made by the mother of a 15-month-old child, reflects a need for further evaluation?

1. "My child takes vitamins everyday."
2. "My child consumes about a liter of milk in a day."
3. "My child's table becomes messy during meal time."
4. "My child is gaining around 1 lb a month."

ANSWER
2

POINTERS
- IDA is characterized by a decreased oxygen-carrying capacity of the blood. The condition is usually associated with nutritional deficiency of iron.
- Manifestations include easy fatigability, poor sucking (infants), and chubby but pale babies (milk babies).
- Decreased Hgb and Hct; microcytic, hypochromic RBCs
- Instruct the client to have frequent rest periods.
- Increase iron in the diet (organ meat, egg yolk) as milk is a poor source of iron. Administer oral iron supplements as ordered.

RATIONALE
Breast milk and cow's milk are poor sources of iron. Furthermore, milk products inhibit the absorption of iron, therefore a child who consumes a liter of milk in a day is at risk for developing iron deficiency anemia.

REFERENCE
Nettina, S. M. (2007). *The Lippincott manual of nursing practice* (8th ed., Philippine ed.). Philadelphia: Lippincott Williams & Wilkins.

NCLEX-RN CATEGORY **Physiological Adaptation**

CONCEPT

Beta blockers trigger bronchospasm.

QUESTION

Which of the following manifestations indicate an adverse effect of beta blockers?

1. Euphoria
2. Wheezing
3. Increased libido
4. Increased appetite

POINTERS

Common side effects of beta blockers

- Impotence
- Decreased libido
- Arrhythmias
- Emotional depression
- Anorexia

ANSWER

2

RATIONALE

Wheezing is indicative of bronchospasm, an adverse effect of beta blockers.

REFERENCE

Karch, A. M. (2007). 2008 *Lippincott's nursing drug guide*. Philadelphia: Lippincott Williams & Wilkins.

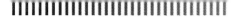

CONCEPT

When on a low-sodium diet, avoid:

Processed foods
Milk products
Salty foods

POINTERS

- The objective of a low sodium diet is to rid the body of excess sodium and fluid accumulation.
- It is used in the treatment of liver disease, renal disease, and hypertension.
- Instruct the client to avoid preservatives, flavor enhancers, and fast food meals.
- Toothpaste, tooth powders, and mouthwashes contain large amounts of sodium.

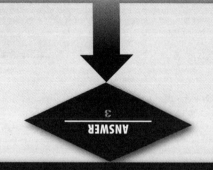

QUESTION

Which of the following foods are allowed for a client on a low-sodium diet?

1. Canned fruits, iced tea, frozen pears
2. Green salad, orange juice, instant soup
3. Tea, chicken sandwich, vegetable salad
4. Bacon and cheese sandwich, fresh fruits, cola

ANSWER

3

RATIONALE

The foods contained in option 3 exclude foods that are high in sodium.

REFERENCE
Dudek, S. G. (2006). *Nutrition essentials for nursing practice* (5th ed.). Philadelphia: Lippincott Williams & Wilkins.

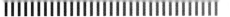

SUBJECT Informed Consent

36

CONCEPT

Emancipated minors can sign a consent form.

POINTERS

- An informed consent protects the client, the surgeon, and the hospital.
- For an unconscious client, permission is required from a responsible member of the family.
- In an emergency situation, witnessed permission by way of telephone is acceptable.
- Emancipated minors (married, with a child, living away from home, in military service) can sign a consent form.
- Procedures that require entry of equipment into a body cavity (bronchoscopy, cystoscopy, colonoscopy) require the client's informed consent.

QUESTION

A 15-year-old adolescent, who delivered a baby boy a month ago, comes to the hospital with the baby for a routine check up. During physical assessment, the physician identifies the presence of a congenital defect in the baby that requires immediate surgery. Which of the following actions is appropriate? The physician:

1. Asks the adolescent's parent to sign the consent
2. Allows the adolescent to sign the consent
3. Refers the situation to the hospital legal committee
4. Defers the surgery

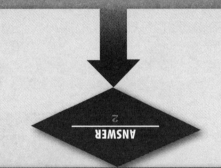

ANSWER

2

RATIONALE

A 15-year-old adolescent with a child is considered an emancipated minor and is therefore legally allowed to sign a consent form.

REFERENCE

Nettina, S. M. (2007). *The Lippincott manual of nursing practice* (8th ed., Philippine ed.). Philadelphia: Lippincott Williams & Wilkins.

CONCEPT

Establishing a contract realizes a more adult approach in relating with a client.

POINTERS

- A contract provides a structure in the nurse–client relationship.
- It defines specific boundaries, roles, and expectations.
- The nurse should ensure that the client agrees with the contract. Noncompliance with the rules may delay discharge of the client.

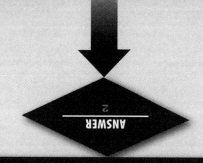

QUESTION

Which of the following nursing actions is the best way to prevent suicide in a depressed client?

1. Frequent scheduled rounds
2. Establishing a "no-self-harm" contract
3. Restraining the client immediately upon admission
4. Keeping the client in an isolation room

ANSWER

2

RATIONALE

Establishing a "no-self-harm" contract enables the nurse to employ a more adult approach in addressing the behavioral problem of a suicidal client.

REFERENCE

Keltner, N. L., Bostrom, C. E., & Schweke, L. H. (2006). *Psychiatric nursing* (5th ed.). Philadelphia: Mosby.

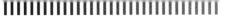

SUBJECT Transcultural Nursing

CONCEPT

Clients from Middle Eastern countries usually prefer to have same-gender healthcare providers because of extreme modesty.

POINTERS

- The religion of Islam traces its origin in Arabia in the 7th century.
- It is considered the world's third largest monotheistic religion.
- The followers of Islam are called Muslims or Moslems.
- Muslims pray 5 times a day while facing east.
- Their diet is called "Halal" (meaning "foods which are allowed").
- Foods which are forbidden are called "Haram."
- Pork is NOT allowed.
- Fasting is done during Ramadan from sunrise to sunset.
- Sick Muslim clients are exempted from fasting.

QUESTION

Which of the following factors will the nurse pay particular attention to when assigning a healthcare provider to a client from a Middle Eastern country?

1. Age
2. Civil status
3. Height and weight
4. Gender

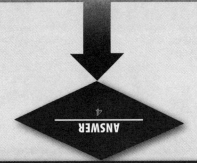

ANSWER

4

RATIONALE

Middle Easterners belong to a male-dominated society. The gender of the healthcare provider affects the degree to which information is revealed by the client.

REFERENCE

Gapuz, R. *The ABCs of passing foreign nursing exams*. Philippines: Gapuz Publications.

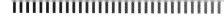
CONCEPT

Open-ended questions are more therapeutic than close-ended questions.

POINTERS

Open-ended questions are those that can be answered in a variety of ways.

Close-ended questions limit the client's answer to either "yes" or "no."

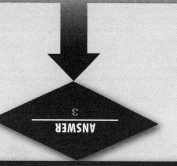

QUESTION

Which of the following questions is appropriate to ask a client with diabetes mellitus?

1. "Do you have any complaints?"
2. "Are you frequently tired?"
3. "How do you clean your feet?"
4. "Do you feel thirsty all the time?"

ANSWER

3

RATIONALE

The question in option 3 is open-ended and is therefore more therapeutic than the close-ended questions.

REFERENCE

Keltner, N. L., Bostrom, C. E., & Schweke, L. H. (2006). *Psychiatric nursing* (5th ed.). Philadelphia: Mosby.

NCLEX-RN CATEGORY **Psychosocial Integrity**

CONCEPT

A positive Guthrie test indicates decreased metabolism of phenylalanine, leading to phenylketonuria.

POINTERS

- The urine PKU test is normally done after 4 to 6 weeks of age.
- If the tests are positive, a blood phenylalanine test is performed.
- Factors that interfere with the results:
  - ▸ Feeding problems
  - ▸ Intake of drugs (aspirin, antibiotics, salicylates)
  - ▸ Prematurity
  - ▸ Lack of protein intake

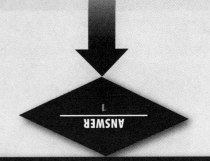

QUESTION

A positive Guthrie capillary blood test reflects which of the following?

1. A metabolic disorder
2. A dietary deficiency
3. A traumatic injury
4. A cancerous lesion

ANSWER

1

RATIONALE

A positive Guthrie test indicates presence of phenylketonuria, a metabolic disorder.

REFERENCE

Pagana, K. D., & Pagana, T. J. (2006). *Mosby's diagnostic and laboratory test reference* (8th ed.). St. Louis, MO: Mosby-Year Book, Inc.

CONCEPT

A positive Romberg's test indicates a problem in the cerebellum.

POINTERS

To perform a Romberg's test:

- Instruct the client to stand erect with the feet together, arms at the sides and without support, first with the eyes open and then with the eyes closed.
- Note the client's ability to maintain balance while the eyes are open and while the eyes are closed.
- A positive test results when the client can stand with eyes open but loses her balance with eyes closed.

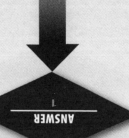

QUESTION

Which of the following interventions is a priority for a client with a positive Romberg's test?

1. Assist the client with ambulation
2. Increase fluid intake of the client to prevent constipation
3. Log-roll the client when transferring him from the bed to a chair
4. Increase fiber in the client's diet

ANSWER

1

RATIONALE

When asked to stand with his feet together and eyes open, the client can maintain the posture, but when asked to close the eyes, the client loses balance. This is a positive Romberg's test. Therefore, the priority is to assist the client with ambulation to prevent falls.

REFERENCE

Nettina, S. M. (2007). *The Lippincott manual of nursing practice* (8th ed., Philippine ed.). Philadelphia: Lippincott Williams & Wilkins.

CONCEPT

Zollinger-Ellison syndrome is characterized by increased gastric hydrochloric acid.

POINTERS

- ZES is due to the presence of a tumor that causes:
  - ▸ Hypersecretion of gastric acids
  - ▸ Duodenal ulcers
  - ▸ Gastrinomas in the pancreas
- ZES is treated with high doses of H2 receptor antagonist
- Octreotide (Sandostatin) is administered to promote suppression of gastric acids.

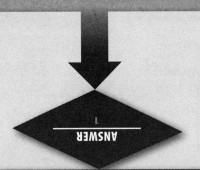

QUESTION

Which of the following findings is common in clients with Zollinger-Ellison syndrome?

1. An elevated hydrochloric acid level
2. Elevated urine specific gravity
3. Elevated serum calcium levels
4. Elevated uric acid levels

ANSWER

1

RATIONALE

An elevated hydrochloric acid level is indicative of Zollinger-Ellison syndrome.

REFERENCE

Nettina, S. M. (2007). *The Lippincott manual of nursing practice* (8th ed., Philippine ed.). Philadelphia: Lippincott Williams & Wilkins.

CONCEPT

Hypertension is a common sign of pheochromocytoma.

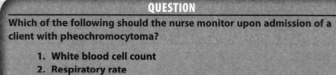

QUESTION

Which of the following should the nurse monitor upon admission of a client with pheochromocytoma?

1. White blood cell count
2. Respiratory rate
3. Hemoglobin level
4. Blood pressure

POINTERS

- Pheochromocytoma is a tumor of the adrenal medulla.
- It is most common between 30 to 60 years of age.
- The presence of the tumor leads to increased production of epinephrine and norepinephrine.
- It is characterized by:

4H
ypertension
ypermetabolism
yperglycemia
eadache

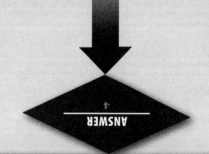

ANSWER

4

RATIONALE

A common sign of pheochromocytoma is hypertension, hence the nurse should monitor the client's blood pressure.

43

NCLEX-RN CATEGORY **Physiological Adaptation**

REFERENCE

Nettina, S. M. (2007). *The Lippincott manual of nursing practice* (8th ed., Philippine ed.). Philadelphia: Lippincott Williams & Wilkins.

44

CONCEPT

Standard precautions must be practiced for all client contacts.

POINTERS

- Standard precautions combine the major features of blood and body fluid precautions and universal precautions.
- It is applied to all clients receiving care in hospitals regardless of their diagnosis or presumed infection status.
- Standard precautions apply to: (1) blood; (2) all body fluids, secretions, and excretions except sweat; (3) nonintact skin; and (4) mucous membranes.
- It entails the use of clean, nonsterile gloves and gown, a mask, eye protection, and a face shield.
- Used needles are not recapped and resuscitation bags are used as alternative to mouth-to-mouth resuscitation in areas where the need for resuscitation is predictable.

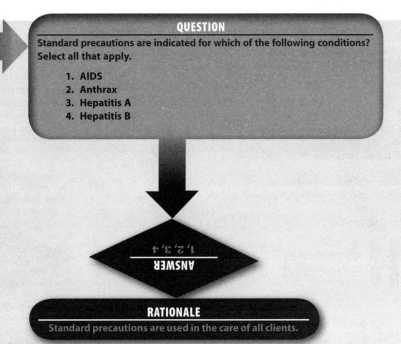

QUESTION

Standard precautions are indicated for which of the following conditions? Select all that apply.

1. AIDS
2. Anthrax
3. Hepatitis A
4. Hepatitis B

ANSWER

1, 2, 3, 4

RATIONALE

Standard precautions are used in the care of all clients.

REFERENCE

Nettina, S. M. (2007). *The Lippincott manual of nursing practice* (8th ed., Philippine ed.). Philadelphia: Lippincott Williams & Wilkins.

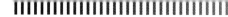
CONCEPT

Utilization of a private room for clients with infectious diseases helps prevent the transfer of infections.

POINTERS

Droplet precaution requirements include a private room, frequent handwashing, and a mask when working within 3 feet of the client.

Droplet precautions are indicated for mycoplasmal pneumonia, streptococcal pharyngitis, scarlet fever, and pertussis.

QUESTION

A client in labor tells the nurse that she had rubella a month ago. Which of the following nursing actions should be a priority after the delivery of the baby?

1. Isolate the baby immediately after delivery
2. Isolate the mother immediately after delivery of the baby
3. Place the client and the baby in a private room
4. Administer rubella vaccines to both the mother and the baby as prescribed

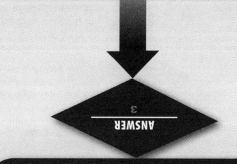

ANSWER

3

RATIONALE

Clients with rubella are placed on droplet isolation precautions, therefore the mother and the baby should be placed in a private room right after delivery.

REFERENCE

Nettina, S. M. (2007). *The Lippincott manual of nursing practice* (8th ed., Philippine ed.). Philadelphia: Lippincott Williams & Wilkins.

NCLEX-RN CATEGORY **Safety and Infection Control**

CONCEPT

Preschoolers should be placed in a room with children belonging to the same age group.

POINTERS

- Preschoolers (ages 4 to 6) are best placed in a room with children belonging to the same age group.
- School-aged children (ages 7 to 12) are best placed in a room with children with the same gender.

QUESTION

Which of the following clients is the best roommate for a 4-year-old child with nephrotic syndrome?

1. A 3-year-old boy with conjunctivitis
2. A 2-year-old girl with laryngotracheobronchitis
3. A 7-year-old boy with fever of unknown origin
4. A 5-year-old girl with fractured tibia

ANSWER

4

RATIONALE

A 5-year-old girl with fractured tibia is non-infectious and therefore could be placed together with a child who has nephrotic syndrome. Preschool children (ages 4 to 6) adapt well if they are placed in a room with a child belonging to the same age group.

REFERENCE

Nettina, S. M. (2007). *The Lippincott manual of nursing practice* (8th ed., Philippine ed.). Philadelphia: Lippincott Williams & Wilkins.

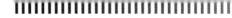
CONCEPT

German measles is transmitted by droplet spread of the virus.

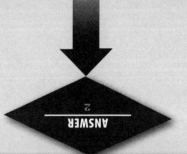

QUESTION

Which of the following equipment is necessary when providing care to a client with German measles?

1. A mask
2. A mask and gloves
3. Gloves and a gown
4. A mask and a gown

ANSWER

2

POINTERS

- The incubation period of rubella is 14 to 21 days.
- Prodromal symptoms like low grade fever, anorexia, headache, and coryza occur first, followed by rubella rash that begins on the face.
- Forscheimer spots (small red petechial macule on the soft palate) may precede or accompany the rash.

RATIONALE

The rubella virus, which causes German measles, is transmitted through contact with the food, urine, stools, and nasopharyngeal secretions of infected persons. It may also be transmitted by contact with contaminated articles of clothing. A mask and gloves are therefore required when providing nursing care.

REFERENCE

Springhouse (Ed.). (2000). *Handbook of infectious diseases*. Philadelphia: Lippincott Williams & Wilkins.

SUBJECT Measles (Rubeola)

CONCEPT

Measles is transmitted by airborne respiratory droplets.

48

POINTERS

- Initial symptoms of measles Include fever, photo phobia, coryza, malaise, anorexia, cough, and hoarseness.
- The hallmark sign is the presence of Koplik's spots.
- Implement airborne precautions.
- The MMR vaccine should not be given to pregnant women, immunosuppressed clients, or clients with an allergy to neomycin.

QUESTION

The measles virus can be transmitted in which of the following manner? Select all that apply.

1. Dust particles
2. Air currents
3. Inhalation
4. Evaporated droplets

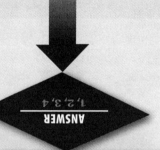

ANSWER
1, 2, 3, 4

RATIONALE

Measles is spread by direct contact or by contaminated airborne respiratory droplets. The portal of entry is the upper respiratory tract.

REFERENCE

Springhouse (Ed.). (2000). *Handbook of infectious diseases*. Philadelphia: Lippincott Williams & Wilkins.

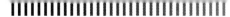

SUBJECT Cryptosporidium Infection

CONCEPT

Cryptosporidiosis is a diarrheal disease transmitted by contaminated water.

POINTERS

- Manifestations of cryptosporidiosis include weight loss, dehydration, fever, nausea, vomiting, and stomach cramps.
- Populations at risk include children who attend daycare centers, travelers, hikers, swimmers, child care workers, and parents of infected children.

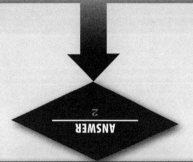

QUESTION

Which data in the client's history increases the risk for cryptosporidium infection?

1. Drinking boiled water from a well
2. Swimming in a public pool
3. Using a water filter with an absolute pore size of 1 micron
4. Peeling raw fruits before eating

ANSWER

2

RATIONALE

Ingestion of food or water contaminated with stool, including water in recreational water parks and swimming pools, is a common mode of transmission of cryptosporidiosis.

49

REFERENCE

Springhouse (Ed.). (2000). *Handbook of infectious diseases.* Philadelphia: Lippincott Williams & Wilkins.

NCLEX-RN CATEGORY **Health Promotion and Maintenance**

SUBJECT Vancomycin Resistant *Staphylococcus aureus* (VRSA)

50

CONCEPT

Clients who are chronically ill or who have a prolonged hospital admission are at risk for VRSA.

POINTERS

- There are no specific signs or symptoms related to VRSA.
- Good handwashing is the most effective way of preventing VRSA.
- Maintain contact precautions.
- Provide a private room and assign equipment for the client's use only.

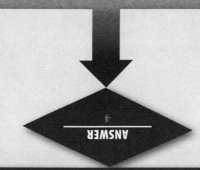

QUESTION

Which of the following clients is least at risk for development of vancomycin resistant *Staphylococcus aureus* (VRSA)?

1. Mary, a 4-year-old with chronic renal failure with an indwelling urinary catheter
2. James, a 35-year-old with cancer of the prostate
3. Jane, a 68-year-old on her third month of hospitalization
4. Mary Jane, a 42-year-old admitted for the first time

ANSWER

4

RATIONALE

A client admitted for the first time has the least risk of developing VRSA because the most at risk populations are those who are chronically ill or who have a prolonged hospital stay or repeated admissions.

REFERENCE

Springhouse (Ed.). (2000). *Handbook of infectious diseases.* Philadelphia: Lippincott Williams & Wilkins.

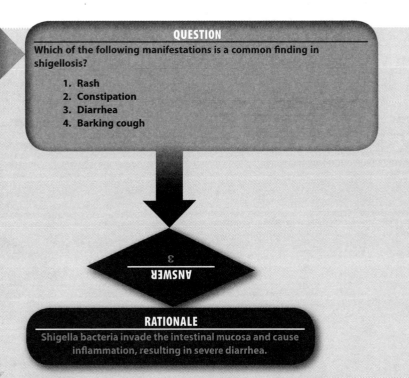

CONCEPT

Shigellosis is characterized by frequent loose watery stools.

POINTERS

- Shigellosis is also known as bacillary dysentery.
- It is transmitted by fecal-oral route.
- Manifestations include high fever and diarrhea with tenesmus.
- PRIORITY: Prevent dehydration.

QUESTION

Which of the following manifestations is a common finding in shigellosis?

1. Rash
2. Constipation
3. Diarrhea
4. Barking cough

ANSWER

3

RATIONALE

Shigella bacteria invade the intestinal mucosa and cause inflammation, resulting in severe diarrhea.

REFERENCE

Springhouse (Ed.). (2000). *Handbook of infectious diseases.* Philadelphia: Lippincott Williams & Wilkins.

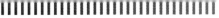

SUBJECT Fourth's Disease (Duke's Disease)

CONCEPT

Duke's disease is a viral rash most commonly caused by enteroviruses.

POINTERS

Manifestations of Duke's disease include fever, nausea, vomiting, diarrhea, photophobia, lymphadenopathy, and sore throat.

QUESTION

The rash in Duke's disease may be characterized as which of the following?

1. Localized with bull's eye pattern
2. Generalized, vesicular, and sometimes petechial
3. Sore spots found in the abdomen
4. Slapped cheek pattern

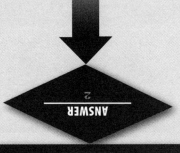

ANSWER

2

RATIONALE

The rash of Duke's disease is characterized as generalized, vesicular, and sometimes petechial.

REFERENCE

Springhouse (Ed.). (2000). *Handbook of infectious diseases.* Philadelphia: Lippincott Williams & Wilkins.

NCLEX-RN CATEGORY Physiological Adaptation

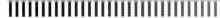

SUBJECT Fifth's Disease

CONCEPT
Fifth's disease is characterized by a "slapped cheek" appearance of rashes.

POINTERS
- Fifth's disease is caused by human parvo virus B 19, and is transmitted via respiratory secretions.
- It is common among children between 4 to 12 years of age and may resolve in about 7 to 10 days.
- Manifestations include a red rash on the cheeks (slapped cheek appearance), low grade fever, malaise, joint pain, and swelling in the hands, wrists, and knees.
- Ig M antibody assay test detects antibody.
- Light and electron microscopy detects B 19 infections to parvo virus.
- Provide frequent rest periods.
- Increase iron in the diet.
- Administer anti-inflammatory medications like aspirin and ibuprofen.
- Implement standard precautions.
- Instruct the client to cover the mouth when coughing or sneezing.

QUESTION
Which of the following statements about Fifth's disease is NOT true?

1. It is transmitted through the respiratory route
2. Polymerase chain reaction detects the presence of the disease
3. It is communicable until the rash develops
4. It is characterized by pruritic rash with desquamation

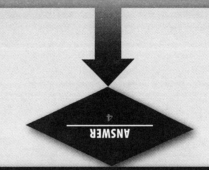

ANSWER
4

RATIONALE
The classic sign of Fifth's disease is erythema on the cheeks (slapped cheek appearance) and a tarry red rash on the trunk and limbs.

53

NCLEX-RN CATEGORY **Physiological Adaptation**

REFERENCE
Springhouse (Ed.). (2000). *Handbook of infectious diseases.* Philadelphia: Lippincott Williams & Wilkins.

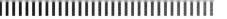

SUBJECT Herpes Zoster

CONCEPT

Severe deep pain occurs in herpes zoster.

POINTERS

Nursing care for clients with herpes zoster

- Primary goal of care is to relieve itching and pain.
- Administer cortisone, tranquilizers, sedatives, tricyclic antidepressants, and acyclovir.
- Apply cold compresses and avoid scratching the lesions.

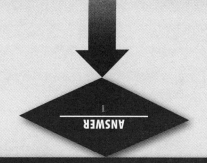

QUESTION

Which of the following is the priority consideration for a client with herpes zoster?

1. Comfort
2. Respiration
3. Mobility
4. Rest

ANSWER

1

RATIONALE

Clients with herpes zoster experience severe deep pain, therefore provision of comfort is a priority consideration.

REFERENCE

Nettina, S. M. (2007). *The Lippincott manual of nursing practice* (8th ed., Philippine ed.). Philadelphia: Lippincott Williams & Wilkins.

NCLEX-RN CATEGORY Physiological Adaptation

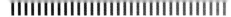

SUBJECT Methicillin-Resistant *Staphylococcus aureus* (MRSA)

CONCEPT
MRSA is transmitted by direct or indirect contact.

QUESTION
Which of the following protective items is/are required when performing colostomy irrigation for a client with methicillin-resistant *Staphylococcus aureus* (MRSA)?

1. Gloves only
2. Gloves and gown
3. Gloves, gown, and goggles
4. Goggles only

POINTERS
- In MRSA, the *Staphylococcus* strain is resistant to methicillin, aminoglycosides, penicillin, cephalosporins and other antibiotics. It usually develops among clients who are using multiple antibiotics as treatment, the elderly, debilitated clients, or clients having multiple invasive procedures.
- Administer vancomycin, the drug of choice, as ordered.
- Place the client in contact precautions.
- Caregiver should wear gowns, masks and gloves.
- Instruct caregivers to cover their mouth and nose when sneezing and coughing.
- Hands must be washed on entering and leaving the room with the use of mild iodine-containing soap.
- Use double bagged method when discarding all articles from the room for disinfection and sterilization.

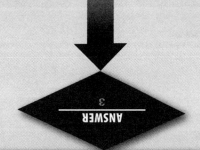

ANSWER 3

RATIONALE
Clients with methicillin-resistant *Staphylococcus aureus* (MRSA) are placed in contact isolation precautions, which include a private room for the client, along with the use of a mask, gown, gloves and goggles.

REFERENCE
Springhouse (Ed.). (2000). *Handbook of infectious diseases.* Philadelphia: Lippincott Williams & Wilkins.

NCLEX-RN CATEGORY Safety and Infection Control

CONCEPT

Histoplasmosis is caused by inhalation of soil contaminated by bat and bird manure.

POINTERS

- Histoplamosis is a fungal infection caused by Histoplasma capsulatum transmitted through ingestion of soil contaminated by bat and bird manure. The incubation period is 5 to 18 days.
- Initially asymptomatic with mild respiratory symptoms, cough, dyspnea, and hemoptysis.
- The clinical manifestations usually resemble tuberculosis.
- Treatment involves antifungal therapy, surgery, and supportive care.
- Administer Fluconazole, Amphotericin B, and steroids as ordered.
- It does not require any isolation precautions. Face mask is worn to prevent ingestion of contaminated soil.
- Refer the client to a social worker and occupational therapist.
- To prevent the occurrence of the disease, instruct the client to avoid going to chicken coops, barns, caves, or under bridges.

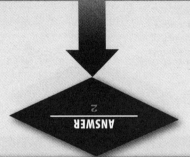

QUESTION

A 10-year-old child who loves to visit the aviary developed cough, fever, dyspnea, and hemoptysis. The nurse should refer the child to the physician for possible treatment of:

1. Tuberculosis
2. Histoplasmosis
3. Sarcoidosis
4. Lyme disease

ANSWER

2

RATIONALE

A child with history of exposure to bird or bat manure with development of cough, fever, dyspnea, or hemoptysis is most likely suffering from histoplasmosis.

REFERENCE

Nettina, S. M. (2007). *The Lippincott manual of nursing practice* (8th ed., Philippine ed.). Philadelphia: Lippincott Williams & Wilkins.

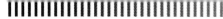

SUBJECT Salmonellosis

CONCEPT
Salmonellosis is associated with intake of soft-boiled eggs or half-cooked meat.

POINTERS
- Salmonellosis is an infection caused by *Salmonella* and is associated with the intake of soft-boiled eggs (egg salad) or half-cooked meat; ingestion of contaminated water; dry milk; chocolate bars; and drugs.
- Stool exam reveals presence of organism.
- Instruct the client to thoroughly cook all eggs and chicken, turkey, and duck meat. Refrigerate meat and foods and avoid keeping them at room temperature for a prolonged period of time.
- Wash hands thoroughly after bowel movement.
- Continue standard precautions until three consecutive stool cultures are negative.
- Report sudden pain in the right lower abdomen, which indicates bowel perforation.

QUESTION
Which of the following is the priority discharge instruction for a client who has been treated for salmonellosis?

1. Keep foods at room temperature
2. Thoroughly cook all eggs and meat
3. Strain the water before using it
4. Do not refrigerate chocolate bars

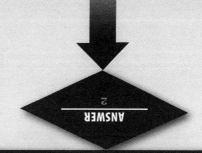

ANSWER 2

RATIONALE
Salmonellosis is associated with the intake of soft-boiled eggs or half-cooked meat, therefore it is important to instruct the client to cook meat and eggs thoroughly.

REFERENCE
Nettina, S. M. (2007). *The Lippincott manual of nursing practice* (8th ed., Philippine ed.). Philadelphia: Lippincott Williams & Wilkins.

NCLEX-RN CATEGORY Physiological Adaptation

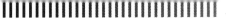

CONCEPT

Rabies virus is transmitted to humans through the saliva of raccoons, dogs, skunks, foxes, and bats.

58

POINTERS

- Rabies is a severe viral infection of the CNS that is communicated to humans by the saliva of infected animals (raccoons, dogs, skunks, foxes, and bats).
- Headache, pruritus, malaise, anorexia, and photophobia develop
- No specific treatment
- Treatment is symptomatic and supportive.
- First aid: wash the bite vigorously with soap and water for at least 10 minutes
- The nurse should wear a gown, gloves, and eye protection when handling saliva and articles contaminated by saliva.
- Confine the suspected animal for 10 days and let it be observed by a veterinarian.
- High risk persons include farm workers, forest rangers, spelunkers (cave explorers), and veterinarians.

QUESTION

Who among the following is most at risk for raccoon bite?

1. Garbage collectors
2. Aviary worker
3. Bus drivers
4. Veterinarians

ANSWER

4

RATIONALE

Farm workers, forest rangers, cave explorers (spelunkers), and veterinarians are at risk for contracting rabies.

REFERENCE

Nettina, S. M. (2007). *The Lippincott manual of nursing practice* (8th ed., Philippine ed.). Philadelphia: Lippincott Williams & Wilkins.

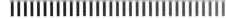

CONCEPT

Sarcoidosis is manifested by fever, night sweats, cough, weight loss, polyarthritis, and mild anemia.

POINTERS

- Sarcoidosis is a chronic, granulomatous multisystem disorder that most notably affects the lungs.
- The exact cause is unknown but the incidence is high in African Americans and young adults.
- Manifestations include fever, night sweats, cough, weight loss, polyarthritis, and mild anemia.
- Diagnosed with KVEIM test: sarcoid node antigen is injected intradermally and causes local nodular lesion in approximately 1 month
- No specific treatment
- Instruct the client to have frequent rest periods.
- Provide small frequent feedings
- Corticosteroids are given to control symptoms.

QUESTION

Which of the following goals of care is appropriate for a client with sarcoidosis?

1. To provide specific treatment
2. To provide frequent rest periods
3. To facilitate bowel elimination
4. To decrease skin irritation

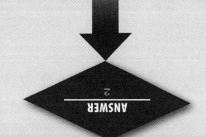

ANSWER
2

RATIONALE

A client with sarcoidosis requires provision of frequent rest periods, because the disease leads to anemia, which causes fatigue.

REFERENCE

Nettina, S. M. (2007). *The Lippincott manual of nursing practice* (8th ed., Philippine ed.). Philadelphia: Lippincott Williams & Wilkins.

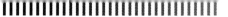
CONCEPT

After admission of a client with bacterial meningitis, the priority goal of care is to prevent the spread of infection.

POINTERS

- Bacterial meningitis is an infection affecting the meninges.
- It is characterized by headache with nuchal rigidity.
- Diagnosed with CSF culture
- Intravenous Penicillin is the drug of choice.
- Implement strict isolation until after the first 24 hours of antibiotic treatment.
- Refer parents of an infected child to an audiologist, because the disease can cause hearing impairment.

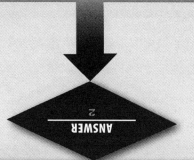

QUESTION

A 6-year-old child with fever, nuchal rigidity, and seizure was admitted. Which of the following is the priority of the nurse upon admission of the child?

1. Assist with feeding
2. Isolate the child
3. Provide a well-lighted room
4. Facilitate bowel elimination

ANSWER

2

RATIONALE

Fever, nuchal rigidity, and seizure are indicative of bacterial meningitis. The priority intervention is to isolate the child to prevent the spread of infection.

REFERENCE

Nettina, S. M. (2007). *The Lippincott manual of nursing practice* (8th ed., Philippine ed.). Philadelphia: Lippincott Williams & Wilkins.

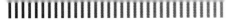

SUBJECT Cohorting

CONCEPT
Clients infected with the same microorganism can share a room.

POINTERS
- A private room is important to prevent direct or indirect contact transmission. It is indicated when the client has poor hygienic practices, a tendency to contaminate the environment, or an inability to maintain infection control precautions (infants, children, clients with altered level of consciousness).
- When a private room is not available, clients infected with the same microorganism can share a room.
- When determining client placement, consider the epidemiology and mode of transmission of the infecting pathogen.

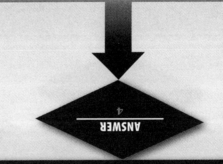

QUESTION
Due to a sudden increase in admission, a private room is not available for a client with tuberculosis. The nurse should therefore place the client in which of the following rooms?

1. Room 112 with a client suffering from diarrhea
2. Room 301 with a client suffering from tuberculosis and rotavirus
3. Room 408 with a client suffering from measles
4. Room 505 with a client suffering from tuberculosis

ANSWER
4

RATIONALE
A client with tuberculosis can be placed in a room together with a client with the same diagnosis.

REFERENCE
Nettina, S. M. (2007). *The Lippincott manual of nursing practice* (8th ed., Philippine ed.). Philadelphia: Lippincott Williams & Wilkins.

NCLEX-RN CATEGORY Safety and Infection Control

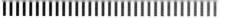

CONCEPT

Clients with complications should be assessed first.

POINTERS

- Bleeding is a danger sign in pregnancy.
- Uterine tenderness and dark vaginal bleeding indicate **abruptio placenta**.
- A boggy uterus with bright red vaginal bleeding indicates **placenta previa**.

QUESTION

Which obstetrical client should the nurse assess first?

1. A 25-year-old class II cardiac client with dyspnea and ankle edema
2. A 27-year-old client with pre-term labor and intact membranes
3. A 30-year-old multiparous post-cesarean client who delivered 3 days ago
4. A 35-year-old client on her 36th week of gestation reporting uterine tenderness and dark vaginal bleeding

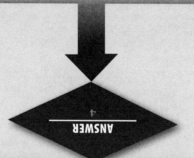

ANSWER

4

RATIONALE

A client on her 36th week of gestation with uterine tenderness and dark vaginal bleeding is possibly suffering from abruptio placenta, which is a complication of pregnancy.

REFERENCE

Pillitteri, A. (2006). *Maternal and child health nursing* (5th ed.). Philadelphia: Lippincott Williams & Wilkins.

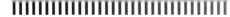

SUBJECT Manifestations of Pregnancy

CONCEPT

Presumptive manifestations of pregnancy include subjective data while probable manifestations include objective findings.

POINTERS

Presumptive manifestations

Amenorrhea
Breast changes
Color changes (face, abdomen, vagina)

Quickening
Nausea and vomiting
Urinary frequency

Probable manifestations

Braxton Hicks contraction
Ballottement
Blood and urine laboratory tests
Fetal outline felt by examiner
Hegar's sign
Goodell's sign

QUESTION

Which of the following manifestations of pregnancy are considered presumptive symptoms? Select all that apply.

1. Amenorrhea
2. Hegar's sign
3. Chloasma
4. Chadwick's sign
5. Striae gravidarum
6. Goodell's signs
7. Frequent urination
8. Positive pregnancy test
9. Fatigue
10. Leukorrhea

63

ANSWER

1, 3, 5, 7, 9

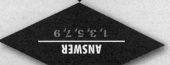

RATIONALE

Presumptive symptoms suggest, but do not prove pregnancy. These include: amenorrhea, breast changes, chloasma/melasma, linea nigra, striae gravidarum, nausea and vomiting, urinary frequency, and fatigue.

REFERENCE

Nettina, S. M. (2007). *The Lippincott manual of nursing practice* (8th ed., Philippine ed.). Philadelphia: Lippincott Williams & Wilkins.

NCLEX-RN CATEGORY **Health Promotion and Maintenance**

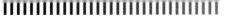

SUBJECT Kegel's Exercises

CONCEPT
Kegel's exercises strengthen the vaginal muscles.

POINTERS
- Kegel's exercises strengthen the pubococcygeal muscle.
- Teach the client to tighten the muscles of the pelvic floor by stopping the flow of urine while urinating and then releasing the muscle to restart the flow.
- Instruct the client to perform 15 contractions in the morning and afternoon and 20 at night or to perform the exercises for 10 minutes, 3 times a day.

NCLEX-RN CATEGORY Health Promotion and Maintenance

QUESTION
Which of the following is the primary purpose of Kegel's exercises in a post-partum client?

1. To promote uterine contraction
2. To strengthen the pelvic muscles
3. To prevent urinary tract infection
4. To prevent urinary incontinence

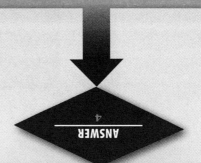

ANSWER
4

RATIONALE
Urinary incontinence is usually due to weakened vaginal muscles. Kegel's exercises will help prevent incontinence by strengthening the vaginal muscles.

REFERENCE
Pillitteri, A. (2006). *Maternal and child health nursing* (5th ed.). Philadelphia: Lippincott Williams & Wilkins.

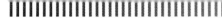

SUBJECT Danger Signs of Pregnancy

CONCEPT

Vaginal bleeding is a danger sign of pregnancy.

POINTERS

Danger signs of pregnancy

Abdominal or chest pain
Bleeding
Chills and fever
Decrease in fetal movement
Escape of clear fluid that suddenly occurs from the vagina
Frequent and persistent vomiting
Gain in weight of over 2 lbs per week in the second trimester or 1 lb per week in the third trimester
Hypertension

PRIORITY

• Report to the physician immediately

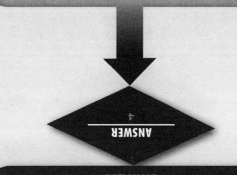

QUESTION

Which of the following clients should the nurse plan to visit first?

1. A post-cesarean multipara who plans to breastfeed
2. A primipara client complaining of abdominal pain that radiates to the back
3. A class II cardiac client complaining of difficulty of breathing after cleaning the house
4. A 36-week gestation client reporting bright red vaginal staining

ANSWER

4

RATIONALE

Vaginal bleeding is a danger sign of pregnancy hence a client who reports bright red vaginal staining should be assessed first.

REFERENCE

Nettina, S. M. (2007). *The Lippincott manual of nursing practice* (8th ed., Philippine ed.). Philadelphia: Lippincott Williams & Wilkins.

NCLEX-RN CATEGORY **Management of Care**

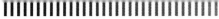

CONCEPT
Report danger symptoms of pregnancy to a healthcare provider.

POINTERS

Danger symptoms of pregnancy

Chills, fever, or burning during urination
Headache
Edema of the face, finger, or sacrum
Visual disturbances
Epigastric pain
Vaginal bleeding
Inability to tolerate foods
Muscular irritability or convulsions

NCLEX-RN CATEGORY Reduction of Risk Potential

QUESTION

Which of the following manifestations, if noted in a pregnant client, needs to be reported to the physician?

1. Hemoglobin of 11 mg/dL
2. Double vision
3. Nausea and vomiting in the morning
4. Amenorrhea

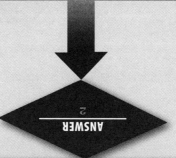

ANSWER

2

RATIONALE

Double vision in a pregnant client is indicative of severe preeclampsia, one of the complications in pregnancy that requires immediate intervention.

REFERENCE

Pillitteri, A. (2006). *Maternal and child health nursing* (5th ed.). Philadelphia: Lippincott Williams & Wilkins.

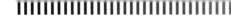

CONCEPT

Pitocin causes retention of water.

POINTERS

- Pitocin is an oxytocic and is used to induce labor after artificial rupture of the membranes
- Causes firmly contracted uterus
- Report the development of rash
- Monitor the BP
- Discontinue if hypertension develops

QUESTION

Which of the following adverse effects occur in prolonged pitocin administration?

1. Labile mood
2. Water intoxication
3. Fever
4. Deep rapid breathing

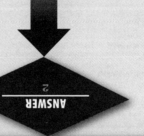

ANSWER

2

RATIONALE

Prolonged administration of Pitocin leads to severe water intoxication.

REFERENCE

Nettina, S. M. (2007). *The Lippincott manual of nursing practice* (8th ed., Philippine ed.). Philadelphia: Lippincott Williams & Wilkins.

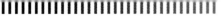

SUBJECT Kleihauer-Betke Test

CONCEPT

A **Kleihauer-Betke test (KB test)** is used to detect fetal-maternal hemorrhage (FMH).

POINTERS

- A KB test is a blood test used to measure the amount of fetal hemoglobin transferred from a fetus to the blood stream of an Rh–negative mother.
- The result of the test can be used to:
  1. Determine the required dose of Rh immunoglobulin to inhibit formation of maternal antibodies.
  2. Prevent Rh disease in future children with Rh-positive blood
- Fetal blood for the test is obtained through the umbilical vein
- Rho immunoglobulin is given to Rh-negative women to prevent sensitization
- Ultrasound is used to monitor for possible bleeding

QUESTION

A Kleihauer-Betke test is performed to help detect which of the following conditions in a client?

1. Neural tube defect
2. Down syndrome
3. Rh incompatibility
4. Sickle cell anemia

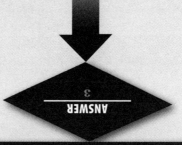

ANSWER

3

RATIONALE

A Kleihauer–Betke test involves examination of blood obtained through the umbilical cord to help detect the presence of Rh incompatibility.

REFERENCE

Pillitteri, A. (2006). *Maternal and child health nursing* (5th ed.). Philadelphia: Lippincott Williams & Wilkins.

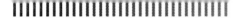

CONCEPT

A reactive NST is characterized by an increase in Fetal Heart Rate (FHR) with fetal movement.

POINTERS

- NST assesses fetal activity and well being.
- A reactive test: an acceleration of fetal heart rate of more than 15 beats per minute above baseline FHR, lasting for 15 seconds or more.
- A non-reactive test: an acceleration of FHR of less than 15 beats per minute above baseline FHR. May indicate fetal jeopardy.

QUESTION

Which of the following findings indicates a reactive non-stress test?

1. FHR remaining unchanged with maternal movement
2. FHR increases with maternal movement
3. FHR increases with fetal movement
4. FHR decreases with fetal movement

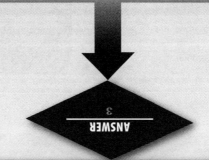

ANSWER

3

RATIONALE

FHR that increases with fetal movement reflects a reactive non-stress test, indicative of an intact central and autonomic nervous system, which is a sign of fetal well-being.

69

NCLEX-RN CATEGORY Reduction of Risk Potential

REFERENCE

Nettina, S. M. (2007). *The Lippincott manual of nursing practice* (8th ed., Philippine ed.). Philadelphia: Lippincott Williams & Wilkins.

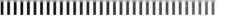

SUBJECT Contraction Stress Test (CST)

CONCEPT

A negative CST result is normal while a positive result is abnormal.

POINTERS

- A negative CST result means an absence of late decelerations.
- A positive CST result means there are persistent late decelerations.
- Persistent late decelerations indicate fetal hypoxia.

QUESTION

Which of the following obstetric clients need to be immediately assessed by the physician?

1. A 30-weeks gestation client with a positive contraction stress test
2. A 32-weeks gestation client with a negative contraction stress test
3. A 12-weeks gestation client who is to undergo a pregnancy test
4. A 34-weeks gestation client who is to undergo a contraction stress test

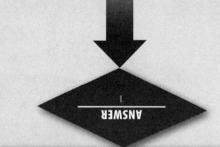

ANSWER

1

RATIONALE

A positive contraction stress test is related to fetal hypoxia, therefore immediate assessment is required.

REFERENCE

Nettina, S. M. (2007). *The Lippincott manual of nursing practice* (8th ed., Philippine ed.). Philadelphia: Lippincott Williams & Wilkins.

CONCEPT

An elevated alpha fetoprotein level (> 30 mg/dL) indicates the presence of neural tube defects.

POINTERS

- A negative contraction stress test indicates that the fetal heart rate remains normal during uterine contraction.
- A positive non-stress test indicates a reactive fetus.
- An increase in glucose in the urine of a pregnant client can be due to accidental spilling of glucose in the urine during pregnancy.

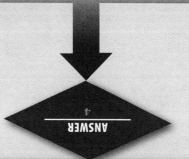

QUESTION

Which of the following diagnostic test results from a pregnant client needs to be reported to the physician immediately?

1. Contraction stress test: Negative
2. Non-stress test: Positive
3. Urinalysis: Increased glucose levels
4. Alpha fetoprotein level: 45 mg/dL

ANSWER

4

RATIONALE

The normal alpha fetoprotein level is 15–30 mg/dL. Elevated levels indicate neural tube defects while decreased levels indicate Down syndrome.

NCLEX-RN CATEGORY **Reduction of Risk Potential**

REFERENCE

Nettina, S. M. (2007). *The Lippincott manual of nursing practice* (8th ed., Philippine ed.). Philadelphia: Lippincott Williams & Wilkins.

CONCEPT

The normal duration of contractions is 30–90 seconds.

POINTERS

Characteristics of uterine contractions

- Mild contractions feel like the tip of the nose.
- Moderate contractions feel like the chin.
- Strong contractions feel like the forehead.
- The normal duration of contractions is 30 to 90 seconds.
- Any contraction that lasts longer than 90 seconds may possibly cause uterine rupture and fetal hypoxia.

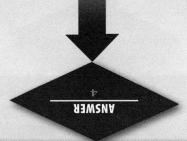

QUESTION

Which of the following client's needs should be assessed first by the nurse?

1. A 30-year-old primigravida in the first stage of labor with regular contractions lasting 30–45 seconds
2. A 20-year-old primigravida in the first stage of labor with regular contractions lasting 45–60 seconds
3. A 25-year-old multigravida in the first stage of labor with two contractions in the last 3 minutes
4. A 27-year-old primigravida in the first stage of labor with three contractions in the last 5 minutes

ANSWER

4

RATIONALE

The presence of only three contractions in 5 minutes indicate that the average duration of each contraction is 100 seconds, which is beyond the normal duration.

REFERENCE

Nettina, S. M. (2007). *The Lippincott manual of nursing practice* (8th ed., Philippine ed.). Philadelphia: Lippincott Williams & Wilkins.

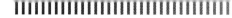

CONCEPT

Labor progresses at a faster rate in a multipara than in a primipara.

POINTERS

- The labor process in a primipara usually lasts for 12 to 15 hours, while in a multipara it is usually 7 to 8 hours.

Danger signs of labor

Abnormal pulse (more than 100 bpm in the mother; and a FHR of above 160 or below 120 in the fetus)

Blood pressure changes (BP above 140/90)

Contour that is abnormal in the lower abdomen (indicates a full bladder which can impede fetal head descent)

QUESTION

Which of the following clients should the nurse bring immediately to the delivery room?

1. A 36-year-old primipara with 7 cm dilatation, fetus at station 0, and intact membranes
2. A 25-year-old primipara with regular contractions every 2 minutes lasting 60–90 seconds with 8 cm dilatation
3. A 28-year-old multipara with 8 cm dilatation and regular contractions occurring every 2–3 minutes lasting 45–60 seconds
4. A 21-year-old primipara with 9 cm dilatation and regular contractions occurring every 5 minutes

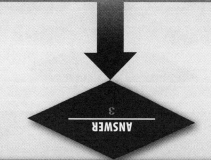

ANSWER
3

RATIONALE

A multipara should be brought to the delivery room when the cervical dilatation is about 8–9 cm.

REFERENCE

Nettina, S. M. (2007). *The Lippincott manual of nursing practice* (8th ed., Philippine ed.). Philadelphia: Lippincott Williams & Wilkins.

74

CONCEPT

True labor contractions are located mainly in the back, occur at regular intervals with increased intensity, and result in progressive cervical dilatation.

POINTERS

Assessment of uterine contractions

Duration refers to the time from the beginning to the end of the same contraction.

Frequency refers to the time from the beginning of the first contraction to the beginning of the next contraction.

Interval refers to the time from the end of the first contraction to the beginning of the next contraction.

QUESTION

Which of the following characteristics of contractions are found in clients with true labor contractions? Select all that apply.

1. Contractions occur at regular intervals
2. Interval between contractions increases
3. Intensity of contractions decreases
4. Contractions are located mainly in the groin
5. Contractions are unaffected by walking
6. Contractions are relieved by mild sedation
7. Contractions do not lead to effacement
8. Contractions occur at irregular intervals
9. Intensity of contractions remains the same
10. Contractions result in progressive cervical dilatation

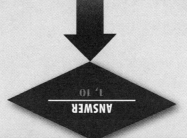

ANSWER 1, 10

RATIONALE

Contractions that occur at regular intervals and are associated with progressive cervical dilatation are characteristics of true labor.

REFERENCE

Pillitteri, A. (2006). *Maternal and child health nursing* (5th ed.). Philadelphia: Lippincott Williams & Wilkins.

SUBJECT Ritodrine (Yutopar)

CONCEPT

Yutopar relaxes the uterus.

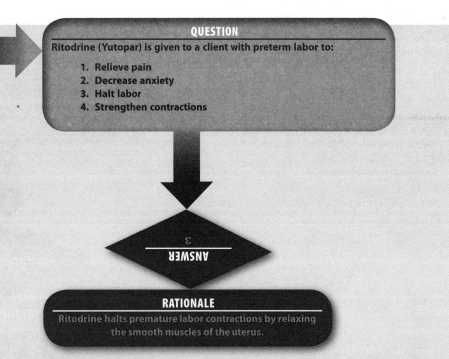

QUESTION

Ritodrine (Yutopar) is given to a client with preterm labor to:

1. Relieve pain
2. Decrease anxiety
3. Halt labor
4. Strengthen contractions

POINTERS

- Yutopar is a tocolytic used to treat preterm labor by decreasing the intensity and frequency of uterine contractions.
- Report an increase in pulse rate; Yutopar causes palpitation.
- Yutopar is contraindicated before the 20th week of pregnancy and in clients with hemorrhage, hypertension, infection, bleeding disorders, and spontaneous abortion.

ANSWER

3

RATIONALE

Ritodrine halts premature labor contractions by relaxing the smooth muscles of the uterus.

REFERENCE

Karch, A. M. (2007). *2008 Lippincott's nursing drug guide*. Philadelphia: Lippincott Williams & Wilkins.

75

NCLEX-RN CATEGORY **Pharmacological and Parenteral Therapies**

CONCEPT

Proper positioning prevents SHS.

76

POINTERS

- SHS is due to the compression of the venous return to the heart by the large uterus
- PRIORITY: Position the client on the left lateral recumbent position

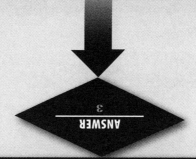

QUESTION

Which of the following interventions is the highest priority for a client with supine hypotensive syndrome (SHS)?

1. Refer the client to the physician at once
2. Assess the client's blood pressure every 2 to 4 hours
3. Place the client on her left side
4. Place the client in Trendelenburg position

ANSWER

3

RATIONALE

Cardiac output increases by 25–30% with an increase in uterine flow when the woman turns from her back to a lateral position, thereby preventing supine hypotensive syndrome.

REFERENCE

Nettina, S. M. (2007). *The Lippincott manual of nursing practice* (8th ed., Philippine ed.). Philadelphia: Lippincott Williams & Wilkins.

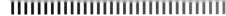

SUBJECT Multiple Myeloma

CONCEPT

Multiple myeloma is a malignant disorder of plasma cells that leads to extensive bone loss, increasing the risk for fractures.

POINTERS

Manifestations of Multiple Myeloma

Pain
Anemia
Insufficient renal function
Neuplastic plasma cell proliferation

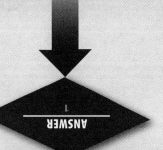

QUESTION

Which of the following nursing diagnoses is a priority for a client with multiple myeloma?

1. Risk for injury
2. Fear
3. Altered tissue perfusion
4. Ineffective breathing pattern

ANSWER

1

RATIONALE

Multiple myeloma can lead to extensive bone loss due to the osteoclast-activity factor (OAF) produced by the plasma cells. This bone loss will eventually result in pathologic fractures, putting the client at risk for injury.

REFERENCE

Nettina, S. M. (2007). *The Lippincott manual of nursing practice* (8th ed., Philippine ed.). Philadelphia: Lippincott Williams & Wilkins.

CONCEPT

The volume of lochia is assessed by noting peri-pad saturation.

POINTERS

Classification of peri-pad saturation

- Less than 1 inch stain: Scant
- 1 inch to less than 4 inches stain: Light
- 4 inches to less than 6 inches stain: Moderate
- Saturated within 1 hour: Heavy

QUESTION

When assessing the lochial discharge of a postpartum client, the nurse notes that the peri-pad has become fully saturated in one hour. This indicates that the lochial discharge is:

1. Scant
2. Light
3. Moderate
4. Heavy

ANSWER

4

RATIONALE

A fully saturated peri-pad in one hour indicates heavy lochial discharge.

REFERENCE

Nettina, S. M. (2007). *The Lippincott manual of nursing practice* (8th ed., Philippine ed.). Philadelphia: Lippincott Williams & Wilkins.

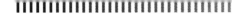

SUBJECT Perineal Hematoma/Postpartum Hematoma

CONCEPT

Pain in the perineal area during the postpartum period indicates perineal hematoma.

POINTERS

Manifestations of Perineal Hematoma

Complaints of pressure and pain
Absence of lochial flow
Possible decrease in blood pressure
Skin that is discolored and painful to touch (first sign)

QUESTION

Which of the following assessment findings in the perineal area of a postpartum client increases the suspicion of a perineal hematoma?

1. Edema
2. Redness
3. Severe pain
4. Warmth

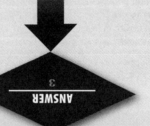

ANSWER

3

RATIONALE

The hematoma causes pressure in the perineal area resulting in severe perineal pain.

REFERENCE
Pillitteri, A. (2006). *Maternal and child health nursing* (5th ed.). Philadelphia: Lippincott Williams & Wilkins.

NCLEX-RN CATEGORY Health Promotion and Maintenance

CONCEPT

UTI increases the incidence of preterm labor.

QUESTION

After the discharge of a client who is 35 weeks gestation following treatment of acute pyelonephritis, the discharge instruction should focus on the signs and symptoms of:

1. Preterm labor
2. Polyhydramnios
3. Polyuria
4. Congestive heart failure

POINTERS

- Preterm labor is characterized by uterine contractions occurring after 20 weeks gestation but before 37 weeks gestation.
- Risk factors include multiple gestation, maternal bleeding, medical conditions like placenta previa, or maternal age of less than 20 years old or greater than 35 years old.

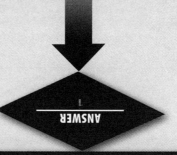

ANSWER

1

RATIONALE

A gravid client with acute pyelonephritis should be advised to watch out for signs and symptoms of preterm labor because urinary tract infections predispose the client to preterm labor.

REFERENCE

Nettina, S. M. (2007). *The Lippincott manual of nursing practice* (8th ed., Philippine ed.). Philadelphia: Lippincott Williams & Wilkins.

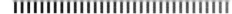

CONCEPT

VBAC is NOT allowed if there is cephalopelvic disproportion.

POINTERS

Criteria for VBAC*

- No documented cephalopelvic disproportion
- Previous cesarean incision was low transverse
- Readily available physician for trial labor
- Emergency surgical facilities are available
- Fetus is less than 4,000 grams (8 lbs, 13 oz)

*Source: American College of Obstetricians and Gynecologists. (2004). Vaginal birth after previous cesarean delivery. ACOG Practice Bulletin, No. 54.

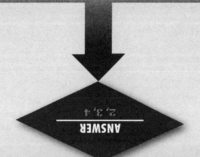

QUESTION

Which of the following condition/s must be present for a client to qualify for a vaginal birth after a previous cesarean delivery? Select all that apply.

1. Cephalopelvic disproportion
2. Previous low transverse cesarean section
3. Presence of stand-by medical personnel
4. Baby's weight is less than 4,000 grams

ANSWER

2, 3, 4

RATIONALE

Women who had a previous cesarean birth are allowed to have vaginal delivery if the previous cesarean involved a low transverse uterine incision, if the baby's weight is < 4000 grams, and if there are medical personnel available to monitor the delivery.

NCLEX-RN CATEGORY Health Promotion and Maintenance

REFERENCE

Nettina, S. M. (2007). The Lippincott manual of nursing practice (8th ed., Philippine ed.). Philadelphia: Lippincott Williams & Wilkins.

82

CONCEPT

Avoid intravaginal examination in clients with bleeding disorders.

POINTERS

- In placenta previa, the placenta attaches low in the uterus.
- Painless, bright red vaginal bleeding occurs after the 7th month of pregnancy.
- Ultrasound will show the location of the placenta.
- Immediate bed rest is the priority.
- Administer IV fluids as ordered.
- Do not perform vaginal exams.

QUESTION

Which of the following interventions should a nurse not implement in a client with placenta previa? Select all that apply.

1. Performing a vaginal exam
2. Using intravaginal fetal heart rate monitoring
3. Frequent assessment of maternal heart rate
4. Bed rest with bathroom privileges
5. Administering IV fluids as ordered

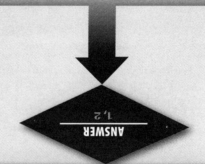

ANSWER

1, 2

RATIONALE

Performing a vaginal exam and using intravaginal fetal heart rate monitoring are contraindicated in clients with placenta previa because these procedures may puncture the placenta.

REFERENCE

Nettina, S. M. (2007). *The Lippincott manual of nursing practice* (8th ed., Philippine ed.). Philadelphia: Lippincott Williams & Wilkins.

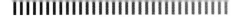

CONCEPT

A common symptom of amniotic fluid embolism is dyspnea.

POINTERS

- Amniotic fluid embolism is a condition in which amniotic fluid escapes into maternal circulation through the placental site into the pulmonary arterioles.
- Dyspnea is the initial manifestation.
- Initiate oxygen therapy as ordered
- Maintain and monitor fluids

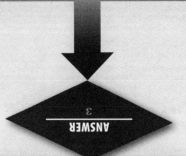

QUESTION

In a client diagnosed to be suffering from amniotic fluid embolism, to which system would the nurse direct his assessment?

1. The nervous system
2. The cardiovascular system
3. The respiratory system
4. The gastrointestinal system

ANSWER

3

RATIONALE

Sudden dyspnea with chest pain after delivery is indicative of amniotic fluid embolism. The nurse should therefore assess the client's respiratory system.

REFERENCE

Nettina, S. M. (2007). *The Lippincott manual of nursing practice* (8th ed., Philippine ed.). Philadelphia: Lippincott Williams & Wilkins.

SUBJECT Disseminated Intravascular Coagulation (DIC)

CONCEPT

The main objective of treatment in DIC is to prevent widespread coagulation all over the body.

POINTERS

- DIC is characterized by widespread coagulation all over the body resulting in a subsequent depletion of clotting factors.
- It is characterized by petechiae and ecchymosis on the skin, mucous membrane, heart, lungs, and other organs.
- Monitor for signs of bleeding (tarry stool, hemoptysis, and nosebleeding).
- Administer Heparin as ordered.
- Heparin inhibits thrombin, thus preventing further clot formation and allowing coagulation factors to accumulate.
- Administer blood transfusion as ordered.
- Instruct the client to avoid aspirin or aspirin-containing compounds.

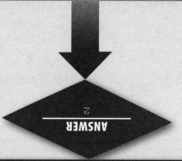

QUESTION

Which of the following is the priority goal of care for a client with disseminated intravascular coagulation?

1. To prevent bleeding
2. To prevent clot formation
3. To avoid aspirin
4. To prolong the bleeding time

ANSWER 2

RATIONALE

In DIC, widespread coagulation all over the body results in a subsequent depletion of clotting factors, which leads to severe hemorrhage. Therefore, to prevent bleeding, the widespread clotting should be prevented.

REFERENCE

Nettina, S. M. (2007). *The Lippincott manual of nursing practice* (8th ed., Philippine ed.). Philadelphia: Lippincott Williams & Wilkins.

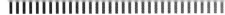
CONCEPT

Bleeding is a common sign of HELLP syndrome.

POINTERS

Manifestations of HELLP syndrome

Hemolysis
Elevated
Liver enzymes
Low
Platelets

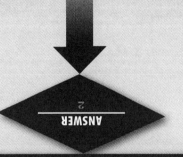

QUESTION

Which of the following assessment findings indicate the development of HELLP syndrome?

1. Decreased ALT and AST
2. Petechiae on the extremities
3. Nausea, anorexia, and vomiting
4. Abdominal and joint pain

ANSWER

2

RATIONALE

Presence of petechiae on the client's extremities is indicative of the development of HELLP syndrome.

REFERENCE

Nettina, S. M. (2007). *The Lippincott manual of nursing practice* (8th ed., Philippine ed.). Philadelphia: Lippincott Williams & Wilkins.

86

CONCEPT

Meconium-stained amniotic fluid in a nonbreech presentation suggests fetal distress.

POINTERS

Signs and symptoms of fetal distress

- Increase or decrease in intensity or frequency of fetal movement (FHR above 160 or below 120 beats per minute)
- Meconium-stained fluid
- Variable or late deceleration pattern

PRIORITY: Position mother to the left side and administer oxygen

QUESTION

Which of the following statements made by a client in labor reflects a need for further evaluation?

1. "I had a greenish discharge when my water broke."
2. "I've had a backache for a couple of hours now."
3. "My baby keeps moving."
4. "My contractions come and go."

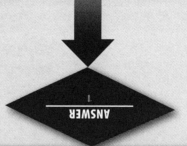

ANSWER

1

RATIONALE

"I had a greenish discharge when my water broke" is indicative of meconium-stained fluid, which is reflective of fetal distress.

REFERENCE

Nettina, S. M. (2007). *The Lippincott manual of nursing practice* (8th ed., Philippine ed.). Philadelphia: Lippincott Williams & Wilkins.

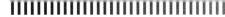

SUBJECT Raloxifene (Evista)

CONCEPT
Evista causes hot flashes.

POINTERS
Keys to safety when giving EVISTA:
- Arrange for periodic blood counts during therapy
- Monitor for possible bleeding
- Administer without regard to food
- Avoid getting pregnant while taking the drug

Common side effects include:
- Hot flashes
- Headache
- Depression
- Vaginal bleeding

Report weakness, sleepiness, mental confusion, pain or swelling of the legs, shortness of breath, or blurred vision to the physician.

QUESTION
Which of the following instructions should the nurse include in the teaching plan for a client receiving raloxifene (Evista)?

1. "It can be taken during pregnancy."
2. "It should always be taken on an empty stomach."
3. "Stay in a place with cool temperatures."
4. "It's all right to take it with cholestyramine."

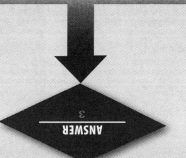

ANSWER
3

RATIONALE
A client who is receiving Evista should be instructed to stay in a place with cool temperatures because the drug causes hot flashes.

REFERENCE
Karch, A. M. (2007). *2008 Lippincott's nursing drug guide*. Philadelphia: Lippincott Williams & Wilkins.

NCLEX-RN CATEGORY Pharmacological and Parenteral Therapies

CONCEPT

Norplant capsules are usually placed under the skin of a woman's upper arm.

POINTERS

- Norplant capsules are placed under the skin of a woman's upper arm.
- It can prevent pregnancy for at least 5 years
- It can cause changes in menstrual bleeding, headache, breast tenderness, acne, weight gain, hair loss, or more hair growth on the face.
- It is effective within 24 hours after insertion.

QUESTION

Which area of the body is the usual site used for implantation of Norplant? Please mark with an X.

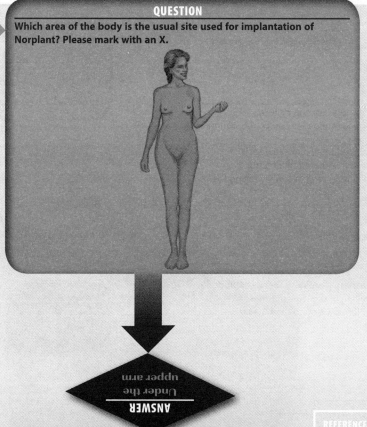

ANSWER

Under the upper arm

RATIONALE

Norplant is inserted in the midportion of the upper arm about 8–10 cm above the elbow crease.

REFERENCE

Karch, A. M. (2007). *2008 Lippincott's nursing drug guide*. Philadelphia: Lippincott Williams & Wilkins.

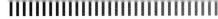

SUBJECT Hydroxyzine (Vistaril)

CONCEPT

Vistaril is used in the first stage of labor to decrease nausea and vomiting.

POINTERS

- Vistaril is an anti-anxiety, antihistamine, and anti-emetic.
- Avoid activities requiring alertness as the drug causes dizziness
- Avoid alcohol, sedatives, and sleep aids
- Encourage frequent oral care to decrease dry mouth
- Report difficulty of breathing, tremors, loss of coordination, sore muscles, or muscle spasms to the physician

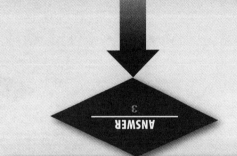

QUESTION

A decrease in which of the following signs and symptoms indicates a positive response to hydroxyzine (Vistaril) for a client in the first stage of labor?

1. Blood pressure
2. Sedation and rest
3. Nausea and vomiting
4. Seizure

ANSWER

3

RATIONALE

Vistaril has an anti-emetic effect that decreases nausea and vomiting in a client in labor.

NCLEX-RN CATEGORY **Pharmacological and Parenteral Therapies**

REFERENCE
Karch, A. M. (2007). *2008 Lippincott's nursing drug guide.* Philadelphia: Lippincott Williams & Wilkins.

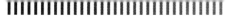

CONCEPT

Pitocin stimulates uterine contraction.

QUESTION

Pitocin is given to a client after delivery of the placenta in order to:

1. Relax the uterus
2. Increase the blood pressure
3. Help control bleeding
4. Prevent thrombophlebitis

POINTERS

- Pitocin is an oxytocic used to induce labor after artificial rupture of the membranes
- It causes contraction of the uterus
- Report the development of a rash
- Monitor the BP
- Discontinue if hypertension develops

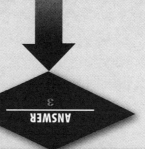

ANSWER

3

RATIONALE

Pitocin reduces postpartum bleeding after expulsion of the placenta by stimulating uterine contractions.

REFERENCE

Karch, A. M. (2007). *2008 Lippincott's nursing drug guide.* Philadelphia: Lippincott Williams & Wilkins.

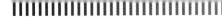

SUBJECT Postpartum Assessment

CONCEPT

A positive Homan's sign should be reported to the physician because it indicates thrombophlebitis.

POINTERS

Postpartum assessment should focus on the following:

- **B**reast
- **U**terus
- **B**ladder
- **B**owels
- **L**ochia
- **E**pisiotomy
- **R**esponse (emotional)
- **S**igns of thrombophlebitis

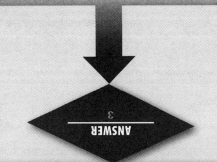

QUESTION

After delivery, which of the following assessment findings in a client should the nurse immediately report to the physician?

1. Bright red vaginal discharge
2. After-pains
3. Pain on dorsiflexion of the leg
4. Leukocytosis

ANSWER

3

RATIONALE

Pain on dorsiflexion of the leg is a positive Homan's sign indicative of thrombophlebitis, which requires prompt assessment and intervention.

REFERENCE

Pillitteri, A. (2006). *Maternal and child health nursing* (5th ed.). Philadelphia: Lippincott Williams & Wilkins.

CONCEPT

A negative statement made by a postpartum client about the infant may suggest difficulty coping.

92

POINTERS

Manifestations of postpartum depresssion

Withdrawal from family
Insomnia
Loss of interest in activities
Lactation difficulties

Decreased sexual responsiveness, dysmenorrhea
Ineffective coping
Exaggerated and prolonged moodiness

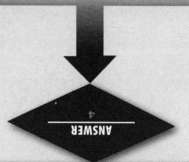

QUESTION

Which of the following statements, if made by a postpartum client, indicates a need for further evaluation?

1. "I don't think I will have enough milk for my baby."
2. "I usually have after pains when I breastfeed my baby."
3. "I will never forget my birthing experience."
4. "The baby isn't as cute as I expected."

ANSWER

4

RATIONALE

The mother's statement, "The baby isn't as cute as I expected", reflects a loss of interest toward her baby, which is indicative of postpartum depression.

REFERENCE

Nettina, S. M. (2007). *The Lippincott manual of nursing practice* (8th ed., Philippine ed.). Philadelphia: Lippincott Williams & Wilkins.

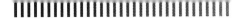

CONCEPT

Weight loss of 5 to 10% of the birth weight is normal in the first two weeks of life.

POINTERS

Normal characteristics of the newborn

Apnea of less than 20 seconds
Breathing that is abdominal and irregular
Cyanosis of the distal extremities (acrocyanosis)

QUESTION

Which of the following assessment findings is considered normal?

1. 25 seconds of apnea
2. Pallor
3. Jaundice in the first 24 hours
4. Weight of 2,700 grams in the second week, down from 3,000 grams at birth

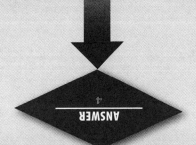

ANSWER

4

RATIONALE

The weight loss of 300 grams falls within the acceptable range of weight loss for neonates, which is 5 to 10% of the birth weight.

REFERENCE

Nettina, S. M. (2007). *The Lippincott manual of nursing practice* (8th ed., Philippine ed.). Philadelphia: Lippincott Williams & Wilkins.

94

CONCEPT

The primary concern in a preterm newborn is the immaturity of all body systems.

POINTERS

Characteristics of preterm newborns

Protective function interference
Resistance to infection is low
Elimination problems
Temperature regulation → unstable
Etiology → placental factors, uterine factors
Respiratory difficulty
Mortality causes:
- Pneumonia
- Septicemia
- Diarrhea
- Meningitis
- Respiratory depression

QUESTION

Which of the following are signs of a premature newborn? Select all that apply.

1. Poor sucking
2. Dry, cracked skin
3. Thin skin
4. Long fingernails
5. Diminished bowel sounds

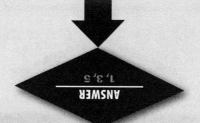

ANSWER

1, 3, 5

RATIONALE

Poor sucking ability, thin skin, and diminished bowel sounds are signs indicative of prematurity in the newborn.

REFERENCE

Pillitteri, A. (2006). *Maternal and child health nursing* (5th ed.). Philadelphia: Lippincott Williams & Wilkins.

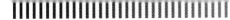

CONCEPT

Introduce one food per week to the infant.

POINTERS

When introducing solid foods to infants, follow this sequence:
- ► Cereals
- ► Fruits
- ► Vegetables
- ► Meat
- ► Table foods
- Cereal is usually given first at 4 months and can be given as a supplement until 18 months.
- Foods are usually introduced one at a time with a 5- to 7-day interval between new foods.
- The infant may be able to hold the spoon and play with it at 9 to 10 months but will not be able to use it for eating until 2 to 3 years old.

QUESTION

Which of the following statements of a mother of an infant indicates a need for further instruction from the nurse?

1. "I'll give 2 to 3 food choices to my child to provide alternatives."
2. "I can begin giving cereals at 4 months."
3. "Milk is a poor source of iron."
4. "I expect my child to be able to use spoon for eating at age 2 to 3."

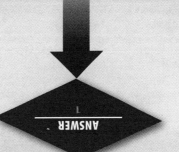

ANSWER
1

RATIONALE

The statement "I'll give 2 to 3 food choices to my child to provide alternatives" requires further health teaching. Ideally, the mother should introduce one food at a time, waiting 5–7 days between new items.

REFERENCE

Pillitteri, A. (2006). *Maternal and child health nursing* (5th ed.). Philadelphia: Lippincott Williams & Wilkins.

CONCEPT

Toys that stimulate the senses are best for infants.

QUESTION

Which of the following toys is appropriate for a 1-month-old child?

1. Brightly colored mobiles
2. Pat-a-cake play
3. Rattle
4. Tricycle bike

POINTERS

Appropriate toys for children

1 month old	→ brightly colored mobile
4 months old	→ rattle
10 months old	→ pat-a-cake or peek-a-boo
Toddlers	→ transportation toys like tricycle
Preschoolers	→ group play like housekeeping toys

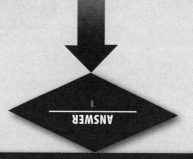

ANSWER

1

RATIONALE

A bright-colored mobile stimulates the senses of the infant.

REFERENCE

Pillitteri, A. (2006). *Maternal and child health nursing* (5th ed.). Philadelphia: Lippincott Williams & Wilkins.

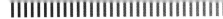

SUBJECT MMR Vaccine

CONCEPT

MMR is made up of live attenuated virus vaccine inoculated from duck eggs.

POINTERS

Contraindications to immunization

- Pregnancy
- Immunosuppression
- Immunodeficiency

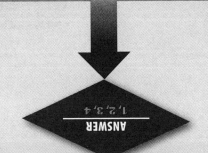

QUESTION

Which of the following questions should the nurse ask the caregiver of a child who is about to receive the MMR vaccine? Select all that apply.

1. "Is the child allergic to eggs?"
2. "Is there anyone in your house having chemotherapy?"
3. "Is there a family member who is immunocompromised?"
4. "Is the child allergic to neomycin?"
5. "Is the child allergic to baker's yeast?"

ANSWER

1, 2, 3, 4

RATIONALE

The nurse should assess for any history of hypersensitivity to neomycin, immune deficiency conditions, allergy to eggs and chicken, or presence of active infection prior to MMR administration.

REFERENCE

Karch, A. M. (2007). *2008 Lippincott's nursing drug guide*. Philadelphia: Lippincott Williams & Wilkins.

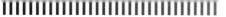

CONCEPT

Dehydration has a more severe effect on infants because their body weight is close to 80% water.

POINTERS

Degrees of dehydration

Mild—less than 5% weight loss
Moderate—5% to 10% weight loss
Severe—more than 10% weight loss

PRIORITY: Maintain hydration

QUESTION

After initial triage, the following clients were referred to the nurse. Which client should the nurse attend to first?

1. An 80-year-old female with no tears while moaning and crying due to abdominal cramps
2. A 7-year-old boy with two episodes of diarrhea in the last hour
3. An 8-month-old baby with three episodes of diarrhea in the last hour
4. A 3-week-old infant with no tears while crying

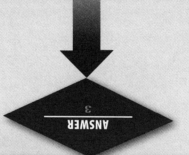

ANSWER
3

RATIONALE

An 8-month-old baby with three episodes of diarrhea in the last hour is at risk for dehydration because their body water approaches 80% of body weight while an average adult has 60%.

REFERENCE

Nettina, S. M. (2007). *The Lippincott manual of nursing practice* (8th ed., Philippine ed.). Philadelphia: Lippincott Williams & Wilkins.

CONCEPT

Drowning is a common cause of accidental death among toddlers.

QUESTION

Which of the following discharge instructions should a nurse provide the parents of a toddler?

1. Begin toilet training when the child reaches 5 years old
2. Do not leave the child near a bucket of water
3. Ignore the child's bedtime rituals
4. Expect the child to be able to ride a bicycle

POINTERS

Talk to the child in simple terms
Offer choices to the child to provide some control
Do not leave alone near the bathtub or swimming pool
Doubt and Shame vs. Autonomy
Learns about death beginning at age 3
Elimination patterns (toilet training begins at 15 to 18 months)
Rituals and routines are common

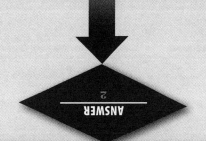

ANSWER

2

RATIONALE

A toddler requires supervision when in a bathtub or near water (including buckets of cleaning water or a washing machine) because drowning is a common cause of accidental death among this age group.

REFERENCE
Pillitteri, A. (2006). *Maternal and child health nursing* (5th ed.). Philadelphia: Lippincott Williams & Wilkins.

NCLEX-RN CATEGORY Safety and Infection Control

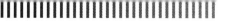

CONCEPT

The best place to auscultate the apical pulse is at the point of maximum impulse.

POINTERS

Apical pulse monitoring

- Place the client in a supine position.
- Ensure that the room is quiet.
- Use the diaphragm of the stethoscope to auscultate the apical area.
- Note that the location of the heart sounds do not correspond to the anatomic location of the valves within the chest.

NCLEX-RN CATEGORY Health Promotion and Maintenance

QUESTION

When obtaining an apical pulse, the best area to place the stethoscope is on the:

1. 2nd intercostal space, right sternal border
2. 2nd intercostal space, left sternal border
3. 5th intercostal space, midclavicular line
4. 5th intercostal space, midaxillary line

ANSWER

3

RATIONALE

The point of maximum impulse is located on the 5th intercostal space, midclavicular line.

REFERENCE

Smeltzer, S. C., Bare, B. G., Hinkle, J. L., & Cheever, K. H. (2006). *Brunner and Suddarth's textbook of medical-surgical nursing.* Philadelphia: Lippincott Williams & Wilkins.

CONCEPT

Restlessness in the neonate indicates hypoxia.

POINTERS

- Acrocyanosis in the newborn is due to premature peripheral circulation.
- Apnea of 5 to 15 seconds decreases with time.
- Newborns sleep for 20 hours a day and feed 6 to 8 times a day.
- Meconium is usually passed in 24 hours.
- Bowel elimination occurs an average of 6 stools per day in the first week.
- Voiding occurs within the first 24 hours.
- Voiding occurs an average of 10 to 15 times a day.
- Tremors and jitteriness indicate hypoxia.

QUESTION

Which infant in the newborn nursery is in need of priority nursing intervention?

1. A 10-hour-old baby with no bowel movement yet
2. A 6-hour-old baby with cyanosis of the hands and feet
3. A 2-hour-old baby with 15 second periods of apnea
4. A 5-hour-old baby with tremors and jitteriness

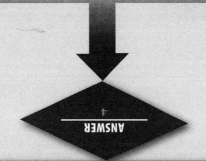

ANSWER

4

RATIONALE

Tremors and jitteriness in the newborn indicate hypoxia, requiring prompt assessment and intervention.

REFERENCE

Pillitteri, A. (2006). *Maternal and child health nursing* (5th ed.). Philadelphia: Lippincott Williams & Wilkins.

101

NCLEX-RN CATEGORY **Management of Care**

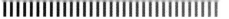
CONCEPT

Mongolian spots are bluish discolorations on the buttocks found in dark-skinned babies.

QUESTION

Mongolian spots are usually found in babies born from which of the following ethnic groups? Select all that apply.

1. East Asian
2. Hispanic
3. East African
4. Native American

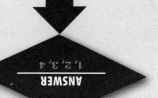

ANSWER

1,2,3,4

POINTERS

- Mongolian spots are irregular areas of deep blue pigmentation in the sacral and gluteal areas in the lower back of newborns of Asian, African, Hispanic, Southern European, and Native American descent.
- The spots may fade as the child reaches 5 years of age.

RATIONALE

Mongolian spots tend to occur in children of Asian, Southern European, Hispanic, African, or Native American descent.

REFERENCE

Pillitteri, A. (2006). *Maternal and child health nursing* (5th ed.). Philadelphia: Lippincott Williams & Wilkins.

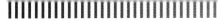
CONCEPT
Anything unusual in an infant should be reported to the physician immediately.

POINTERS
Unusual occurrences in the infant

- Salty skin → cystic fibrosis
- Apathy → cretinism
- Bleeding after circumcision → hemophilia
- Bleeding after tooth extraction → Von Willebrand's disease
- Apnea of more than 20 seconds → apnea of infancy
- Early pattern of hand dominance (before 10–12 months) → cerebral palsy
- Currant-jelly stool (mucoid with blood) → intussusception
- Jaundice in the first 24 hours after delivery → pathologic jaundice

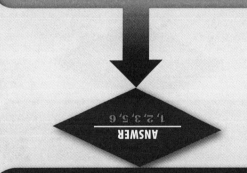

QUESTION
Which of the following statements made by a mother regarding her baby need to be reported to the physician? Select all that apply.

1. "My baby tastes salty."
2. "My baby seldom cries."
3. "My baby had bleeding after circumcision."
4. "Sometimes, my baby doesn't breathe for as long as 10 seconds."
5. "I discovered at 7 months that my child is left-handed."
6. "My baby's stool is mucoid and bloody."
7. "I don't know whether my baby will ever get his teeth; he still doesn't have any at 5 months."

ANSWER
1, 2, 3, 5, 6

RATIONALE
The statements indicate the presence of abnormalities in infants.

REFERENCE
Nettina, S. M. (2007). *The Lippincott manual of nursing practice* (8th ed., Philippine ed.). Philadelphia: Lippincott Williams & Wilkins.

NCLEX-RN CATEGORY **Reduction of Risk Potential**

104

CONCEPT

Gower's sign is present when a client uses the upper extremities to brace the body as he attempts to stand.

POINTERS

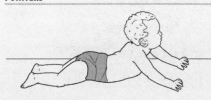

- Gower's sign is indicative of a genetically transmitted muscular disorder.

QUESTION

The nurse is obtaining the history of a client with Duchenne's muscular dystrophy. Which of the following motor skills is initially affected by the disorder?

1. Deep breathing
2. Sitting
3. Standing
4. Swallowing

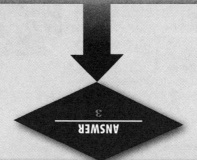

ANSWER
3

RATIONALE

The hallmark feature of Duchenne's muscular dystrophy is characterized by a child's difficulty in standing. A client with Duchenne's muscular dystrophy uses the upper extremities to brace the body as he attempts to stand.

REFERENCE
Springhouse (Ed.). (2006). *Professional guide to signs and symptoms* (5th ed.). Philadelphia: Lippincott Williams & Wilkins.

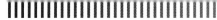

SUBJECT Crepitus

CONCEPT

Crepitus is found in clients with subcutaneous emphysema.

POINTERS

How to assess for crepitus:

Subcutaneous emphysema
- A crackling, grating sound in the thorax may be heard by auscultation.

Fractures
- A grating sensation can be felt

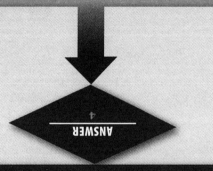

QUESTION

How should the nurse assess for crepitus in a client with subcutaneous emphysema?

1. Palpation
2. Percussion
3. Inspection
4. Auscultation

ANSWER

4

RATIONALE

When assessing for crepitus, a grating, crackling sound can be heard upon auscultation of the affected area.

REFERENCE

Smeltzer, S. C., Bare, B. G., Hinkle, J. L., & Cheever, K. H. (2006). *Brunner and Suddarth's textbook of medical-surgical nursing.* Philadelphia: Lippincott Williams & Wilkins.

CONCEPT

The priority intervention in hypoxemia is to administer oxygen.

POINTERS

Manifestations of hypoxemia

- Progressive changes in mental status
- Dyspnea
- Increased blood pressure
- Diaphoresis
- Cool extremities
- Central cyanosis (late sign)

PRIORITY: Administer oxygen as prescribed

QUESTION

A 35-year-old male client has a decreased level of consciousness. The client's PaO_2 is 61% and the $PaCO_2$ is 55%. Based on this information, which nursing action is of highest priority?

1. Provide instructions on pursed-lip breathing
2. Initiate chest physiotherapy
3. Connect the client to pulse oximetry
4. Administer oxygen as prescribed

ANSWER

4

RATIONALE

Administration of oxygen is the highest priority nursing action in clients with hypoxemia.

REFERENCE

Nettina, S. M. (2007). *The Lippincott manual of nursing practice* (8th ed., Philippine ed.). Philadelphia: Lippincott Williams & Wilkins.

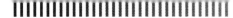
CONCEPT

Intermittent claudication refers to calf pain that is worsened by activity and relieved by rest.

POINTERS

- Measures to relieve intermittent claudication include smoking cessation, walking and range of motion exercise, and avoidance of crossing legs while sitting.
- Report any of the following to the physician:
  Bruises and blisters
  Redness and swelling
  Itching
  New areas of ulceration

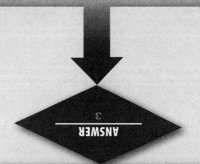

QUESTION

How should the nurse assess for intermittent claudication?

1. Ask the client to stand up and close his eyes
2. Ask the client to smoke a cigarette and then cough
3. Ask the client to walk until he complains of pain and then allow him to rest
4. Ask the client to flex and extend the lower extremities

ANSWER

3

RATIONALE

To assess for the presence of intermittent claudication, the nurse should instruct the client to walk until he complains of pain and then allow him to rest.

107

NCLEX-RN CATEGORY Physiological Integrity

REFERENCE

Nettina, S. M. (2007). *The Lippincott manual of nursing practice* (8th ed., Philippine ed.). Philadelphia: Lippincott Williams & Wilkins.

CONCEPT

Ginkgo biloba can cause bleeding.

POINTERS

- Ginkgo biloba improves blood circulation.
- Contraindications include pregnancy, lactation, and clotting disorders.
- Monitor:
  ▸ RR, HR, PT, PTT
- Uses:
  Dementia (Alzheimer's disease)
  Intermittent claudication
  PMS
  Diabetic retinopathy
  Altitude sickness
  Tinnitus
- Side effects:
  ▸ Severe side effects are rare
  ▸ Headache
  ▸ Dizziness
  ▸ Heart palpitations
  ▸ GI reactions
  ▸ Rash (resembles poison ivy)

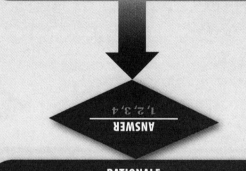

QUESTION

A client who is scheduled for knee surgery in two weeks is being interviewed by the nurse. Which of the following herbal remedies should the nurse instruct the client to stop taking? Select all that apply.

1. St. John's wort
2. Ginkgo biloba
3. Kava-kava
4. Valerian

ANSWER
1, 2, 3, 4

RATIONALE
These herbal remedies will put the client at risk for bleeding.

REFERENCE
Karch, A. M. (2007). *2008 Lippincott's nursing drug guide*. Philadelphia: Lippincott Williams & Wilkins.

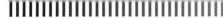

CONCEPT
St. John's wort causes photosensitivity.

POINTERS
St. John's wort

- Monitor vision, PT, PTT, and sleep pattern
- Uses:
  Bronchitis
  Asthma
  Gout

  Depression
  Anxiety
  Rheumatism
  Tonsillitis
  Sciatica

- Side effects:
  ▸ Photosensitivity
  ▸ Rash
  ▸ Tachycardia

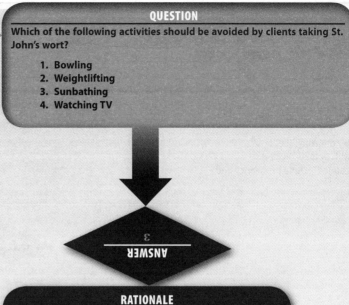

QUESTION
Which of the following activities should be avoided by clients taking St. John's wort?

1. Bowling
2. Weightlifting
3. Sunbathing
4. Watching TV

ANSWER
3

RATIONALE
Clients who are taking St. John's wort may experience photosensitivity and must be instructed to refrain from having too much sun exposure.

REFERENCE
Karch, A. M. (2007). 2008 *Lippincott's nursing drug guide.* Philadelphia: Lippincott Williams & Wilkins.

SUBJECT Saw Palmetto

CONCEPT

Saw palmetto decreases the size of the prostate gland, thereby facilitating urination.

POINTERS

- Saw palmetto stops progression of BPH-like finasteride.
- Eases urinary difficulty
- Interferes with iron absorption
- Contraindications include pregnancy and lactation.
- Uses:
  BPH
  Asthma
  Diuretic
  Cough
  Astringent
  Bronchitis
- Side effects:
  ▶ Headache
  ▶ Diarrhea

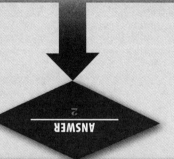

QUESTION

Which of the following symptoms in a client with benign prostatic hypertrophy decreases with the intake of saw palmetto?

1. Headache
2. Dysuria
3. Polyuria
4. Hematuria

ANSWER

2

RATIONALE

Saw palmetto decreases the prostate gland thereby relieving dysuria.

REFERENCE

Springhouse (Ed.). (2005). *Nursing herbal medicine handbook.* Philadelphia: Lippincott Williams & Wilkins.

NCLEX-RN CATEGORY Basic Care and Comfort

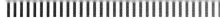

SUBJECT Ginkgo Biloba

CONCEPT
Ginkgo biloba thins the blood.

POINTERS
- Ginkgo biloba improves blood circulation.
- Contraindications include pregnancy, lactation, and clotting disorders.
- Monitor: RR, HR, PT, PTT
- Uses:
  Dementia (Alzheimer's disease)
  Intermittent claudication
  PMS
  Diabetic retinopathy
  Altitude sickness
  Tinnitus
- Side effects:
  ▸ Severe side effects are rare
  ▸ Headache
  ▸ Dizziness
  ▸ Heart palpitations
  ▸ GI reactions
  ▸ Rash (resembles poison ivy)

QUESTION
Ginkgo biloba should not be used by a client who is also receiving which of the following medications? Select all that apply.

1. Coumadin
2. Heparin
3. Aspirin
4. Streptokinase

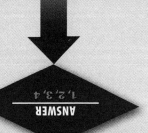

ANSWER 1, 2, 3, 4

RATIONALE
Ginkgo biloba thins the blood. Therefore it should not be given with coumadin, heparin, aspirin, or streptokinase because when taken with ginkgo biloba, these drugs may increase the risk of bleeding.

REFERENCE
Springhouse (Ed.). (2005). *Nursing herbal medicine handbook.* Philadelphia: Lippincott Williams & Wilkins.

NCLEX-RN CATEGORY **Basic Care and Comfort**

SUBJECT Ma Huang

CONCEPT

Ma huang is a central nervous system stimulant.

QUESTION

Which of the following indicates a common effect of ma huang?

1. Fatigue
2. Increased energy level
3. Irritability
4. Severe depression

POINTERS

- Effects of ma huang:
  - ▸ Weight loss
  - ▸ Enhanced energy level
- Withdrawal effects:
  - ▸ Severe depression
  - ▸ Irritability
  - ▸ Fatigue
- Side effects:
  - ▸ **C**ardiac arrythmias
  - ▸ **H**eadache
  - ▸ **I**nsomnia
  - ▸ **N**ervousness
  - ▸ **D**epression (in children)
  - ▸ **D**izziness
- Do not use with MAOI antidepressants; this combination may cause hypertensive crisis.

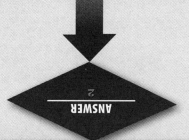

ANSWER

2.

RATIONALE

An increased energy level is a common effect of ma huang because it stimulates the central nervous system.

REFERENCE
Springhouse (Ed.). (2005). *Nursing herbal medicine handbook.* Philadelphia: Lippincott Williams & Wilkins.

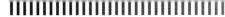

SUBJECT Di Huang

CONCEPT

Di huang is used as an oral treatment for diabetes mellitus.

POINTERS

Di huang is usually given orally to clients with diabetes mellitus to decrease blood sugar levels

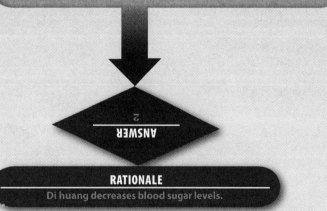

QUESTION

Which of the following assessment parameters indicates the therapeutic effects of di huang?

1. Hemoglobin of 8 mg/dL
2. Blood sugar level of 85 mg/dL
3. Urine-specific gravity of 1.035
4. White blood cell count of 3,500

ANSWER 2

RATIONALE

Di huang decreases blood sugar levels.

REFERENCE

Springhouse (Ed.). (2005). *Nursing herbal medicine handbook*. Philadelphia: Lippincott Williams & Wilkins.

NCLEX-RN CATEGORY **Basic Care and Comfort**

CONCEPT

Echinacea should NOT be used for treatment of autoimmune disorders.

POINTERS

- Echinacea is an immune system stimulant.
- It should not be used for more than 14 days.
- Store it away from direct light.
- Uses:
  - ▸ Upper respiratory tract infection
  - ▸ Urinary tract infection
  - ▸ Eczema
- Contraindicated in progressive disorders such as
  - ▸ Multiple sclerosis
  - ▸ HIV
  - ▸ AIDS

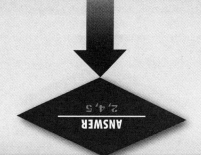

QUESTION

Echinacea is used as a treatment for which of the following conditions? Select all that apply.

1. Systemic lupus erythematosus
2. Flu
3. Multiple sclerosis
4. Urinary infection
5. Toothache

ANSWER

2, 4, 5

RATIONALE

Systemic lupus erythematosus and multiple sclerosis are autoimmune disorders hence echinacea should not be given.

REFERENCE

Springhouse (Ed.). (2005). *Nursing herbal medicine handbook*. Philadelphia: Lippincott Williams & Wilkins.

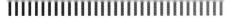

CONCEPT

Black cohosh decreases menopausal symptoms.

QUESTION

A decrease in which of the following manifestations of menopause indicates the effectiveness of black cohosh?

1. Diarrhea
2. Hot flashes
3. Nausea and vomiting
4. Breast tenderness

POINTERS

- Black cohosh is used for the relief of premenstrual discomfort, dysmenorrheal, and menopausal symptoms.
- It does not affect the vaginal epithelium, so it does not relieve vaginal dryness.
- It should not be used for more than 6 months.
- Manifestations of overdose include nausea, vomiting, dizziness, visual disturbance, slowed pulse rate, and increased perspiration.

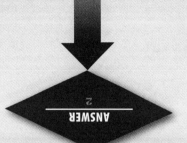

ANSWER

2

RATIONALE

Black cohosh is effective in treating symptoms of menopause, including hot flashes, sweating, sleep disturbance, and anxiety.

REFERENCE

Springhouse (Ed.). (2005). *Nursing herbal medicine handbook.* Philadelphia: Lippincott Williams & Wilkins.

CONCEPT

Kava kava causes coma when combined with alprazolam.

QUESTION

Kava kava is used in the treatment of all of the following conditions except:

1. Nervous anxiety
2. Coma
3. Stress
4. Restlessness

POINTERS

- Uses of kava kava:
  - ▸ Local anesthetic
  - ▸ Sedative
  - ▸ Sleep aid
- Side effects:
  - ▸ Dry, flaking, discolored skin
  - ▸ Scaly rash
  - ▸ Red eyes
  - ▸ Puffy face
  - ▸ Muscle weakness
  - ▸ CNS depression
- Contraindicated in:
  - ▸ Pregnancy
  - ▸ Lactation

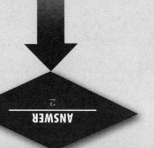

ANSWER 2

RATIONALE

Kava kava affects the limbic system, modulating emotional processes to produce anxiolytic effects. When given together with alprazolam, it causes coma.

REFERENCE

Springhouse (Ed.). (2005). *Nursing herbal medicine handbook.* Philadelphia: Lippincott Williams & Wilkins.

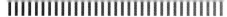

SUBJECT Chamomile

CONCEPT

Chamomile causes bronchospasm.

POINTERS

- Uses of chamomile:
  Cutaneous burn
  Diarrhea
  Stomatitis
- Monitor for menstrual changes and pregnancy
- Tea used in sedation; relaxation
- Side effects:
  ▸ Contact allergies
  ▸ Anaphylaxis (shortness of breath, swelling of the tongue, rash, tachycardia, hypotension)

QUESTION

A client who is receiving theophylline (Theo-dur) should be cautioned not to take which of the following herbal remedies?

1. Chamomile
2. Garlic
3. Gotu kola
4. Ginkgo biloba

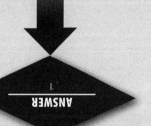

ANSWER

1

RATIONALE

Theophylline causes bronchodilation whereas chamomile causes bronchoconstriction. They are antagonistic and therefore should not be taken at the same time.

NCLEX-RN CATEGORY Basic Care and Comfort

REFERENCE
Springhouse (Ed.). (2005). *Nursing herbal medicine handbook.* Philadelphia: Lippincott Williams & Wilkins.

CONCEPT

Blue cohosh has an oxytocic effect.

POINTERS

Uses of blue cohosh

- Regulation of menstrual cycle
- Eases painful cramps
- Used to jumpstart stalled labor
- Used to stop bleeding

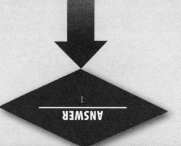

QUESTION

Blue cohosh is commonly used during the last 2–4 weeks of pregnancy in order to:

1. Give the uterus final toning
2. Promote closure of the cervix
3. Regulate menstruation
4. Prevent bleeding

ANSWER

1

RATIONALE

Blue cohosh has an oxytoxic effect, hence it is used during the last few weeks of pregnancy in order to give the uterus final toning.

REFERENCE

Springhouse (Ed.). (2005). *Nursing herbal medicine handbook*. Philadelphia: Lippincott Williams & Wilkins.

CONCEPT

Complete bed rest is indicated for a client with cervical radium implant to prevent the implant from dislodging.

POINTERS

Nursing care of clients with radium implants

Restrict visitors.

Avoid direct contact around the implant site. Observe proper distance and position when providing nursing care depending on the sources of radiation.

Do not touch a dislodged radiation source with bare hands; use long handled forceps. Keep a pair of forceps at the bedside.

Implement strict isolation and radiation precautions.

Organize nursing tasks to minimize exposure to the client (30 minutes per shift is ideal).

Observe for signs of complications like nausea, vomiting, bleeding, or infection.

Note the following:
- ► Pregnant women or individuals less than 18 years old should not be allowed to go inside the client's room.
- ► Visitors should stand 6 feet away from the client.

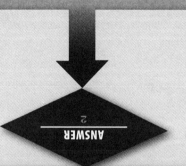

QUESTION

Which of the following instructions is NOT indicated for a client with cervical cancer with a radium implant?

1. Complete bed rest
2. Brief periods of ambulation
3. Assuming a low-Fowler's position
4. Ensuring bladder emptying

ANSWER

2

RATIONALE

Cervical cancer clients with a radium implant require complete bed rest. Allowing the client brief periods of ambulation will potentially cause the radium implant to dislodge.

REFERENCE

Nettina, S. M. (2007). *The Lippincott manual of nursing practice* (8th ed., Philippine ed.). Philadelphia: Lippincott Williams & Wilkins.

CONCEPT

A common risk factor of breast cancer is nulliparity.

POINTERS

Breast cancer risk factors

History in the family
Age
Sex

Benign breast disease
Early menarche
Estrogen replacement therapy (controversial issue)
Nulliparity

Biopsy result indicative of atypical ductal hyperplasia
Advanced age (late menopause)
Diet high in fat

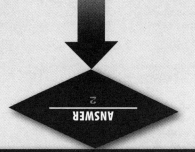

QUESTION

Which of the following statements made by a female client reflects a need for further evaluation?

1. "I had a history of being hit with a ball when I was 9."
2. "I had my first baby when I was 35."
3. "We lived in a house built in the 1960s since I was born."
4. "I make sure that I get my flu shots yearly."

ANSWER

2

RATIONALE

Nulliparity, or having the first child after the age of 30, places the client at risk for breast cancer.

REFERENCE

Nettina, S. M. (2007). *The Lippincott manual of nursing practice* (8th ed., Philippine ed.). Philadelphia: Lippincott Williams & Wilkins.

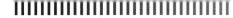
CONCEPT

A change in voice is a common manifestation of laryngeal cancer.

POINTERS

- Laryngeal cancer is characterized by the presence of malignant cells in the larynx. It is associated with smoking and alcoholism.
- Hoarseness, voice change, or a tickling sensation in the throat occurs
- Laryngoscopy and biopsy reveal malignant cells
- Prepare the client for radiation, chemotherapy, and surgery
- Teach client to avoid cold air
- Instruct the client that swimming is not recommended post-laryngectomy.

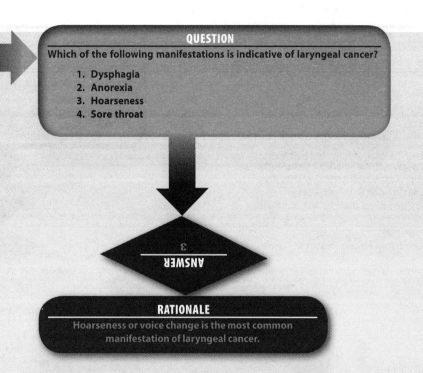

QUESTION

Which of the following manifestations is indicative of laryngeal cancer?

1. Dysphagia
2. Anorexia
3. Hoarseness
4. Sore throat

ANSWER

3

RATIONALE

Hoarseness or voice change is the most common manifestation of laryngeal cancer.

REFERENCE

Gapuz, R. *The ABCs of passing foreign nursing exams*. Philippines: Gapuz Publications.

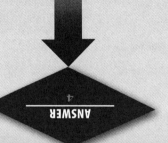

CONCEPT

Zofran decreases nausea and vomiting.

POINTERS

- Zofran prevents nausea and vomiting related to chemotherapy and radio-therapy.
- Best given 30 minutes before chemotherapy
- Report difficulty of breathing after drug administration to the physician
- Drug may cause diarrhea and constipation
- Assess the heart rate; drug may cause arrhythmia
- Monitor liver function tests

QUESTION

Which of the following statements, if made by a client who is receiving ondansetron (Zofran), indicates a positive response to the medication?

1. "I don't have pain anymore."
2. "I'm eating a lot now."
3. "I sleep better now."
4. "I don't feel nauseous anymore."

ANSWER

4

RATIONALE

The statement that the client doesn't feel nauseous anymore indicates that the drug has exerted its therapeutic effect of preventing nausea and vomiting.

REFERENCE

Karch, A. M. (2007). *2008 Lippincott's nursing drug guide*. Philadelphia: Lippincott Williams & Wilkins.

SUBJECT Azathioprine (Imuran)

CONCEPT

Imuran causes immunosuppression.

POINTERS

- Take Imuran with food if gastric irritation occurs
- Avoid going to crowded areas
- Notify the physician immediately when injured
- Common side effects include nausea, vomiting, diarrhea, and skin rash.
- Report episodes of bleeding, bruising, and signs of infection to the physician

QUESTION

Which of the following discharge instructions should the nurse provide a client who is to receive azathioprine (Imuran) after organ transplant?

1. "Monitor your blood pressure frequently."
2. "Avoid going to the market."
3. "The drug may increase urine output."
4. "Fever is a common side effect of the drug and should therefore not be reported to the physician."

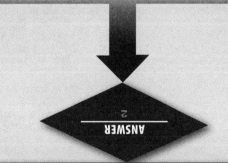

ANSWER

2

RATIONALE

Clients who are immunosuppressed should avoid going to crowded areas.

123

REFERENCE

Karch, A. M. (2007). *2008 Lippincott's nursing drug guide.* Philadelphia: Lippincott Williams & Wilkins.

NCLEX-RN CATEGORY **Health Promotion and Maintenance**

CONCEPT

Adriamycin is cytotoxic.

POINTERS

- Adriamycin is an antineoplastic antibiotic.
- Best taken in the morning
- May turn the urine red, and can cause diarrhea or alopecia
- Increase fluid intake; the drug can cause hyperuricemia
- Assess for allergy

QUESTION

Which of the following statements, if made by a client who is receiving doxorubicin hydrochloride (Adriamycin), would indicate to a nurse that the client needs further instruction about the use of the drug?

1. "I know I will have loose stools."
2. "My heartbeat may become faster."
3. "My urine will turn red."
4. "I will need to limit my fluid intake."

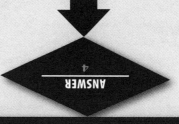

ANSWER

4

RATIONALE

Adriamycin is a cytotoxic drug, therefore the nurse should instruct the client to increase oral fluid intake during the course of therapy.

REFERENCE

Karch, A. M. (2007). *2008 Lippincott's nursing drug guide.* Philadelphia: Lippincott Williams & Wilkins.

CONCEPT

Late stream hematuria is associated with bladder cancer.

POINTERS

- Normal characteristics of urine
  - ▶ Clear
  - ▶ Faint aromatic odor
  - ▶ Yellow or amber
  - ▶ Ph: 4.6 to 8.0
  - ▶ Specific gravity: 1.010 to 1.025
  - ▶ Osmolarity:
    Male: 390 to 1,090 mOsm/kg
    Female: 300 to 1,090 mOsm/kg
- Abnormal characteristics of urine
  - ▶ Cloudy urine → infection
  - ▶ Straw colored → dilute urine
  - ▶ Highly colored/deep amber → concentrated urine, sign of inadequate fluid intake
  - ▶ Smokey colored/dark red → hematuria
  - ▶ Reddish brown → bleeding
  - ▶ Yellow brown or green brown or dark yellow → obstructive jaundice/increased bilirubin levels
  - ▶ Fixed specific gravity at 1.010 → chronic renal failure
  - ▶ Decreased specific gravity (below 1.005) → diabetes insipidus
  - ▶ Increased specific gravity (above 1.030) → diabetes mellitus

QUESTION

Which of the following statements made by a client is indicative of bladder cancer?

1. "My urine turns bloody when I start to urinate."
2. "My urine turns bloody before I end my urination."
3. "My urine is pinkish from the beginning to the end of my urination."
4. "I have had red-orange urine for several weeks now."

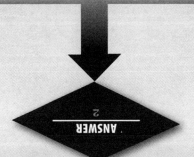

ANSWER

2

RATIONALE

Late stream hematuria, described as bloody urine before the end of urination, is usually associated with bladder lesions. Early stream hematuria is usually associated with urethral lesions.

REFERENCE

Nettina, S. M. (2007). *The Lippincott manual of nursing practice* (8th ed., Philippine ed.). Philadelphia: Lippincott Williams & Wilkins.

CONCEPT

Surgical interventions on the chest and abdominal area may affect respiration.

POINTERS

Post-operative care

- Assess respiratory status
- Auscultate breath sounds to identify respiratory complications
- Encourage turning, coughing, and deep breathing while splinting the incision
- Assist the client with ambulation
- Administer pain medications as prescribed

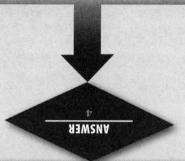

QUESTION

After a splenectomy, which of the following assessments is a nursing priority?

1. The drainage on the client's dressing
2. The client's blood pressure
3. The client's pupillary reaction
4. The quality of the client's respiration

ANSWER

4

RATIONALE

Due to the proximity of the surgical incision to the diaphragm, the initial nursing intervention post-operatively is to assess the airway and maintain adequate respiratory function.

REFERENCE

Nettina, S. M. (2007). *The Lippincott manual of nursing practice* (8th ed., Philippine ed.). Philadelphia: Lippincott Williams & Wilkins.

CONCEPT

Preschoolers usually have loose teeth.

POINTERS

- Recurrent or persistent tonsillitis 4 times a year is an indication for a tonsillectomy.
- Post-operatively, assess for signs of bleeding:
  - ▶ Tachycardia
  - ▶ Frequent swallowing
  - ▶ Pallor
  - ▶ Restlessness
- Keep suction equipment at the bedside
- Offer cool fruit juices, cool water, and popsicles for first 12 to 24 hours

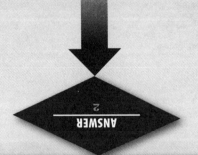

QUESTION

A 6-year-old child is being scheduled for tonsillectomy. Which of these assessment findings needs to be reported to the physician immediately?

1. A history of frequent upper respiratory tract infections
2. The presence of loose teeth
3. A verbalized fear of the unknown and body mutilation
4. A tendency to boast and tell a lie

ANSWER

2

RATIONALE

The presence of loose teeth before administration of anesthesia poses a danger. If the loose teeth get dislodged during the surgical procedure, it may potentially lead to complications.

REFERENCE

Nettina, S. M. (2007). *The Lippincott manual of nursing practice* (8th ed., Philippine ed.). Philadelphia: Lippincott Williams & Wilkins.

CONCEPT

Any condition that interferes with breathing increases the risk for pneumonia.

POINTERS

Nursing care of clients post-cholecystectomy

- Priority: Assess for pain and administer prescribed analgesic to facilitate deep breathing and coughing exercises
- Encourage ambulation to prevent thromboembolism and to stimulate bowel and bladder function
- Instruct the client to keep the incision or wound sites dry for 5 to 7 days
- Report signs of redness, pain, or drainage

QUESTION

Which of the following conditions is a client most at risk for post-cholecystectomy?

1. Tetany
2. Curling's ulcer
3. Hypostatic pneumonia
4. Deep vein thrombosis

ANSWER

3

RATIONALE

The breathing pattern of a post-op client is impaired due to pain, therefore the client becomes unable to clear the airway, which increases the risk for hypostatic pneumonia.

REFERENCE

Nettina, S. M. (2007). *The Lippincott manual of nursing practice* (8th ed., Philippine ed.). Philadelphia: Lippincott Williams & Wilkins.

SUBJECT Fentanyl Transdermal Patch

CONCEPT

Fentanyl acts as an analgesic when applied on the upper torso.

POINTERS

- Prepare the application site by clipping the hair; do not shave
- Apply on dry skin and avoid using lotion
- Patch must be worn continuously for 72 hours
- Side effects:
  - ▶ Sedation
  - ▶ Sweating
  - ▶ Slow shallow respiration
  - ▶ Suppression of cough reflex
  - ▶ Spasm of urinary sphincter
  - ▶ Shock
  - ▶ Sensitivity to cold

QUESTION

Which area of the body is the best site for applying a fentanyl patch? Please mark with an X.

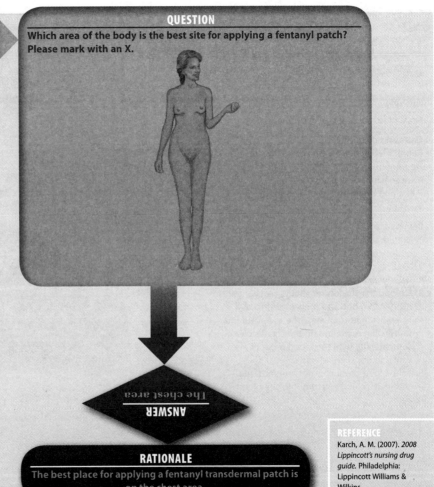

ANSWER

The chest area

RATIONALE

The best place for applying a fentanyl transdermal patch is on the chest area.

REFERENCE

Karch, A. M. (2007). *2008 Lippincott's nursing drug guide*. Philadelphia: Lippincott Williams & Wilkins.

CONCEPT

In treatments requiring venous infusion, STOP the treatment at the first sign of adverse reaction.

POINTERS

Signs of immediate transfusion reaction

Chills and diaphoresis
Rapid thready pulse, rashes
Apprehension
Muscle aches, back pain, chest pain
Pallor and cyanosis
Swelling

Reminders:
1. Note that ONLY normal saline should be added to blood components.
2. Medications are NEVER added to blood transfusions.
3. A blood transfusion set should be changed every 4 to 6 hours to prevent septicemia.
4. The most important step of administering a transfusion is confirming the client's blood compatibility with the blood product and verifying the client identity.
5. If the blood product is not administered within 30 minutes, return it to the blood bank.

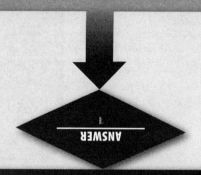

QUESTION

Which of the following nursing actions is the priority of the nurse when a transfusion reaction occurs?

1. Stop the blood transfusion and replace it with normal saline
2. Adjust the blood transfusion rate and monitor the client
3. Monitor the input and output
4. Refer to the physician immediately

ANSWER

1

RATIONALE

At the initial sign of a transfusion reaction, the nurse should immediately discontinue the transfusion and notify the physician.

REFERENCE

Nettina, S. M. (2007). *The Lippincott manual of nursing practice* (8th ed., Philippine ed.). Philadelphia: Lippincott Williams & Wilkins.

CONCEPT

Risk factors for thromboembolism:
- Older adults with fractures
- History of thrombophlebitis
- Immobilized
- Obese

POINTERS

Prevention of thromboembolism

- Encourage active and passive ankle exercises
- Elevate the legs
- Encourage mobility
- Report calf pain and increased calf size and temperature

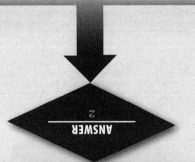

QUESTION

Which of the following clients is most at risk for thromboembolism?

1. A 55-year-old client with osteoporosis
2. A 60-year-old client in traction
3. A 15-year-old adolescent with an inflamed knee
4. A 20-year-old young adult with weight loss

ANSWER

2

RATIONALE

An elderly client who is placed in traction is at high risk for developing thromboembolism because of stasis of blood.

REFERENCE

Nettina, S. M. (2007). *The Lippincott manual of nursing practice* (8th ed., Philippine ed.). Philadelphia: Lippincott Williams & Wilkins.

CONCEPT

A fibrinogen level below 100 mg/dL needs to be reported to the physician.

POINTERS

- Fibrinogen is essential to promote blood clotting.
- Fibrinogen level is used in the diagnosis of bleeding disorders.
- Normal level is 200 to 400 mg/dL.
- A fibrinogen level below 100 mg/dL indicates a bleeding disorder.
- Oral contraceptives and estrogen increase fibrinogen level.
- Anabolic steroids, androgens, asparaginase, phenobarbital, streptokinase, urokinase, and valproic acid decrease fibrinogen level.

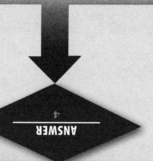

QUESTION

After surgery, which of the following laboratory values would be most critical for the nurse to assess and report to the physician due to the possibility of disseminated intravascular coagulation (DIC)?

1. Prothrombin time (PT) of 14 seconds
2. Hemoglobin level of 13
3. Activated partial thromboplastin time (APTT) of 64 seconds
4. Fibrinogen level of 80 mg/dL

ANSWER

4

RATIONALE

A fibrinogen level below 100 mg/dL must be reported immediately to the physician because it indicates a bleeding disorder.

REFERENCE

Nettina, S. M. (2007). *The Lippincott manual of nursing practice* (8th ed., Philippine ed.). Philadelphia: Lippincott Williams & Wilkins.

NCLEX-RN CATEGORY Reduction of Risk Potential

CONCEPT

A client with iron deficiency anemia will usually complain of:
- Fatigue
- Fainting
- Forgetfulness

POINTERS

- IDA is characterized by decreased oxygen carrying capacity of the blood. The condition is usually associated with a nutritional deficiency of iron.
- Those afflicted have easy fatigability, poor sucking (infants), and chubby but pale babies (milk babies).
- Decreased Hgb and Hct; microcytic, hypochromic RBCs
- Instruct the client to have frequent rest periods.
- Increase iron in the diet (organ meat, egg yolk); milk is a poor source of iron. Administer oral iron supplements as ordered.

QUESTION

Which comment of a client would be indicative of nutritional anemia?

1. "My headache is on and off."
2. "I always feel tired and short of breath."
3. "I have difficulty sleeping at night."
4. "My legs feel weak after a long walk."

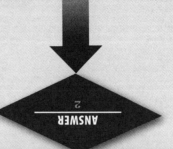

ANSWER

2

RATIONALE

Iron deficiency is caused by an inadequate supply of iron for RBC formation, resulting in decreased oxygen carrying capacity. Therefore, the client will manifest easy fatigability, fainting, and forgetfulness. Other symptoms may include dyspnea on exertion, pallor, and inability to concentrate.

REFERENCE

Nettina, S. M. (2007). *The Lippincott manual of nursing practice* (8th ed., Philippine ed.). Philadelphia: Lippincott Williams & Wilkins.

133

NCLEX-RN CATEGORY Physiological Adaptation

CONCEPT

Cooley's anemia is transmitted by the autosomal recessive pattern of inheritance.

POINTERS

- Beta thalassemia major is an inherited form of anemia characterized by decreased and defective production of hemoglobin.
- It affects people of Italian, Greek, African, Malaysian, and Chinese descent.

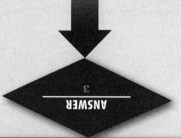

QUESTION

The parents of a child diagnosed with Cooley's anemia should be referred to a/an:

1. Audiologist
2. Endocrinologist
3. Geneticist
4. Physical therapist

ANSWER

3

RATIONALE

Cooley's anemia is a genetically determined, inherited disease through autosomal recessive pattern of inheritance. Therefore the child's parents should be referred to a geneticist for genetic counseling.

REFERENCE

Nettina, S. M. (2007). *The Lippincott manual of nursing practice* (8th ed., Philippine ed.). Philadelphia: Lippincott Williams & Wilkins.

SUBJECT Folic Acid Deficiency Anemia (FADA)

CONCEPT

Folic acid deficiency anemia (FADA) is characterized by hemolytic anemia and exfoliative dermatitis.

POINTERS

- FADA is commonly associated with alcoholism, excessive cooking of food, and malnutrition.
- It is characterized by fatigue, fainting, forgetfulness, sore tongue, and cracked lips.
- Include food sources of folic acid in the diet such as beef, liver, peanut butter, red beans, oatmeal, broccoli, and asparagus.
- Avoid overcooking vegetables.

QUESTION

Which of the following manifestations are indicative of folic acid deficiency anemia? Select all that apply.

1. Pallor
2. Weakness
3. Sore tongue
4. Headache
5. Tachycardia

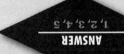

ANSWER

1, 2, 3, 4, 5

RATIONALE

Clinical manifestations of folic acid deficiency related to anemia include fatigue, pallor, weakness, headache, and tachycardia. Other symptoms related to folic acid deficiency include sore tongue and cracked lips.

REFERENCE

Nettina, S. M. (2007). *The Lippincott manual of nursing practice* (8th ed., Philippine ed.). Philadelphia: Lippincott Williams & Wilkins.

CONCEPT

Hemarthrosis or bleeding into the joints is the hallmark sign of hemophilia.

POINTERS

- Hemophilia is due to a deficiency of clotting factors. It is a sex-linked recessive trait (type A and B), and more common in males but transmitted by females. Von Willebrand's disease is transmitted to both male and female offsprings of a carrier.
- There is hemarthrosis (bleeding joints) usually in the elbows, ankles, and knees. Increased pain means bleeding continues.
- Partial thromboplastin time is prolonged but there is normal prothrombin time.
- Avoid aspirin
- Control bleeding by utilizing RICE:
  - **R**est
  - **I**mmobilize
  - **C**old compress (10–15 minutes)
  - **E**levate
- Avoid contact sports and rectal temperature monitoring.
- Administer missing coagulation factors as ordered. Stop transfusion if hives, headache, tingling, chills, flushing, or fever develops.
- Administer short course of corticosteroids to relieve inflammation.
- Refer to physical therapy to prevent contractures and orthotics to prevent joint injury.
- Gentle, passive exercise 48 hours after the acute phase can be implemented for less severe hemarthroses.
- Airway obstruction may occur due to bleeding in the neck and pharynx.

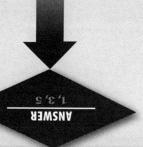

QUESTION

Which of the following joints are usually affected in hemophilia? Select all that apply.

1. Elbows
2. Wrists
3. Knees
4. Distal interphalangeal joints
5. Ankles

ANSWER

1, 3, 5

RATIONALE

Hemorrhages into the joints or hemarthrosis are commonly founds in the elbows, knees, and ankles.

REFERENCE

Nettina, S. M. (2007). *The Lippincott manual of nursing practice* (8th ed., Philippine ed.). Philadelphia: Lippincott Williams & Wilkins.

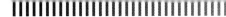

CONCEPT

Aplastic anemia is characterized by pancytopenia.

POINTERS

- Aplastic anemia is due to bone marrow hypoplasia or aplasia resulting in pancytopenia (decreased WBC, RBC, and platelets).
- Prepare the client for a bone marrow transplant
- Assess for signs and symptoms of bleeding

QUESTION

Which of the following blood components are affected in aplastic anemia? Select all that apply.

1. Erythrocytes
2. Leukocytes
3. Thrombocytes
4. Factor IX

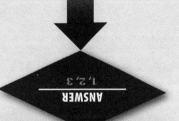

ANSWER
1, 2, 3

RATIONALE

Aplastic anemia is characterized by bone marrow hypoplasia or aplasia resulting in decreased RBCs, WBCs, and platelets. A deficiency in factor IX is associated with hemophilia B or Christmas disease, not with aplastic anemia.

REFERENCE
Nettina, S. M. (2007). *The Lippincott manual of nursing practice* (8th ed., Philippine ed.). Philadelphia: Lippincott Williams & Wilkins.

138

CONCEPT

Polycythemia vera is characterized by increased RBC mass and hemoglobin.

POINTERS

- Manifestations of polycythemia vera:
  Reddish purple hue of skin
  Uric acid formation
  Splenomegaly
  Headache and hepatomegaly
- Treatment includes:
  ▸ Phlebotomy (withdrawal of 250 to 500 ml of blood)
  ▸ Allopurinol, to decrease uric acid levels
  ▸ Antihistamine to decrease pruritus

QUESTION

Which of the following laboratory data are elevated in polycythemia vera? Select all that apply.

1. Hemoglobin
2. Hematocrit
3. Blood glucose
4. Red blood cell count
5. Urine output

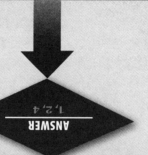

ANSWER

1, 2, 4

RATIONALE

Polycythemia vera is a chronic myelo-proliferative disorder involving all bone marrow elements, resulting in an increase in RBC mass and hematocrit.

REFERENCE

Nettina, S. M. (2007). *The Lippincott manual of nursing practice* (8th ed., Philippine ed.). Philadelphia: Lippincott Williams & Wilkins.

CONCEPT

Appropriate interventions prevent complications.

POINTERS

- To prevent sickle cell crisis, the priority intervention is to promote hydration.
- To prevent dyspnea, a client with myocardial infarction should be given frequent rest periods.
- To prevent lead poisoning, children who are living in houses built in the 1960s should be assessed and the parents referred to housing authorities.

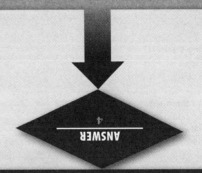

QUESTION

Who among the following clients is at greatest risk for complications?

1. Mrs. Jones, with history of sickle cell anemia, who frequently drinks water
2. Mr. Tad, with history of myocardial infarction, who takes time to sit in between his lectures
3. Nemia, who lives in a neighborhood of houses built in the 1960s
4. Mimi, a 15 weeks age of gestation having pica with ice chips

ANSWER

4

RATIONALE

Pica with ice chips in a pregnant client increases the risk for physiologic anemia.

139

REFERENCE

Nettina, S. M. (2007). *The Lippincott manual of nursing practice* (8th ed., Philippine ed.). Philadelphia: Lippincott Williams & Wilkins.

NCLEX-RN CATEGORY **Reduction of Risk Potential**

CONCEPT

Remember the characteristics of:
Abdominal sounds
Breath sounds
Cardiac sounds

POINTERS

- **A**bdominal sounds are assessed using the diaphragm of the stethoscope. Normal gurgling, high-pitched sounds are heard every 5 to 20 seconds. If the client is hungry, borborygmi or prolonged growling sounds are considered normal.
- **B**reath sounds are auscultated using the diaphragm of the stethoscope. Place the diaphragm directly on the client's skin. Normal breath sounds are identified as vesicular (low pitch and best heard during inspiration), bronchovesicular (best heard in the 1st and 2nd ICS), and bronchial sounds (high pitch and best heard over the trachea).
- **C**ardiac sounds are best heard using the diaphragm of the stethoscope. S1 and S2 are normal cardiac sounds; S3 is normal in children but may indicate heart failure in the elderly.

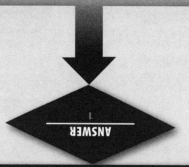

QUESTION

Which of the following sounds auscultated in the different parts of the body is abnormal?

1. Vascular sound in the abdomen
2. Clear breath sounds in the chest
3. S3 sounds in the sternum of a pediatric client
4. Growling sounds in the abdomen

ANSWER

1

RATIONALE

A vascular sound or bruits heard over the abdomen is indicative of abdominal aortic aneurysm. Normally, the abdomen should have a "growling" sound.

REFERENCE

Nettina, S. M. (2007). *The Lippincott manual of nursing practice* (8th ed., Philippine ed.). Philadelphia: Lippincott Williams & Wilkins.

CONCEPT

HBOT involves breathing 100 percent oxygen in a sealed chamber. It is a painless procedure.

POINTERS

HBOT is used for the treatment of:
- Air embolism
- Wounds
- Carbon monoxide poisoning
- Radiation injuries
- Burns

QUESTION

A client who is to undergo hyperbaric oxygen therapy asks the nurse "Is it painful?" The appropriate response of the nurse is:

1. "Yes, it is."
2. "No, although you may feel some fullness in your ears."
3. "There will be prickling sensations."
4. "Yes, but medications will be given to decrease the pain."

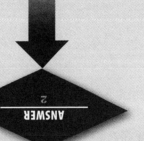

ANSWER

2

RATIONALE

Hyperbaric oxygen therapy is a painless procedure. However, it has potential side effects, including ear trauma, central nervous system disorders, and oxygen toxicity.

141

REFERENCE

Smeltzer, S. C., Bare, B. G., Hinkle, J. L., & Cheever, K. H. (2006). *Brunner and Suddarth's textbook of medical-surgical nursing.* Philadelphia: Lippincott Williams & Wilkins.

NCLEX-RN CATEGORY **Reduction of Risk Potential**

CONCEPT

Xanthopsia is a common manifestation of digoxin toxicity.

POINTERS

Manifestations of digoxin toxicity

- Slow, irregular pulse
- Rapid weight gain
- Loss of appetite
- Nausea
- Vomiting
- Blurred or "yellow" vision
- Weakness
- Swelling of the ankles, legs, or fingers
- Difficulty breathing

PRIORITY:

- Monitor drug therapeutic levels: 0.5 to 2 ng/mL
- Keep digoxin immune fab ready if toxicity occurs

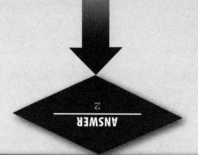

QUESTION

Which of the following statements, if made by a client receiving digoxin (Lanoxin) 0.25 mg daily, needs to be reported to the physician?

1. "I check my pulse rate regularly."
2. "The TV screen doesn't look good to me."
3. "I am having tunnel vision."
4. "My appetite got better."

ANSWER

2

RATIONALE

Xanthopsia, or yellowish green vision, affects the client's field of vision. It is a common sign of digoxin toxicity.

REFERENCE

Karch, A. M. (2007). *2008 Lippincott's nursing drug guide.* Philadelphia: Lippincott Williams & Wilkins.

SUBJECT Potassium Chloride

CONCEPT

Potassium is primarily excreted in the urine.

QUESTION

Before administration of potassium chloride, what should the nurse check?

1. Blood pressure
2. Respiratory rate
3. Temperature
4. Urine output

POINTERS

- Take potassium chloride after meals or with food.
- Do not crush or chew tablets.
- Dissolve liquid form with cold water or juice and drink it slowly.
- Before administration, assess the following:
  ▸ Skin color
  ▸ Baseline ECG
  ▸ Bowel sounds
  ▸ Urine output
  ▸ Serum electrolytes

ANSWER

4

RATIONALE

Potassium should be administered only after adequate urine flow has been established. Potassium is primarily excreted by the kidneys; therefore, when oliguria occurs, potassium administration can cause the serum potassium concentration to rise dangerously.

REFERENCE

Karch, A. M. (2007). *2008 Lippincott's nursing drug guide.* Philadelphia: Lippincott Williams & Wilkins.

NCLEX-RN CATEGORY **Pharmacological and Parenteral Therapies**

SUBJECT Dobutamine Hydrochloride (Dobutrex)

CONCEPT

Dobutamine has a positive inotropic effect.

POINTERS

Common adverse effects of dobutamine

- Headache
- Nausea
- Tachycardia
- Palpitation

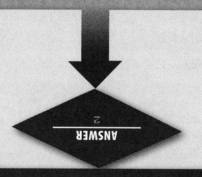

QUESTION

Dobutamine hydrochloride (Dobutrex) is administered to a client with cardiac decompensation in order to:

1. Depress cardiac contractility
2. Increase cardiac output
3. Diminish cardiac output
4. Promote renal retention of fluids

ANSWER

2

RATIONALE

Dobutamine hydrochloride is a B1 selective adrenergic agonist that has a positive inotropic effect, which increases myocardial contractility leading to increased cardiac output.

REFERENCE

Karch, A. M. (2007). *2008 Lippincott's nursing drug guide.* Philadelphia: Lippincott Williams & Wilkins.

CONCEPT

Vitamin K-containing green leafy vegetables counteract the effects of coumadin.

POINTERS

- Coumadin is an anticoagulant and prevents thrombus formation; it does not dissolve clots.
- Avoid green leafy vegetables as the vitamin K content of these vegetables interferes with the absorption of the drug.
- Avoid contact sports.
- Assess for any sign of bleeding.
- Keep vitamin K at the bedside.
- Do not give client any IM injection.
- Many factors (diet, fever, environment) may change the body's response to the drug.

QUESTION

Which of the following foods is allowed for a client who is taking coumadin?

1. Spinach
2. Broccoli
3. Asparagus
4. Wheat bread

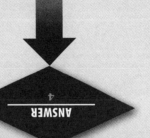

ANSWER

4

RATIONALE

A client who is taking coumadin should avoid eating foods rich in vitamin K, such as green leafy vegetables, because these foods may antagonize the desired effect of the drug.

REFERENCE

Karch, A. M. (2007). *2008 Lippincott's nursing drug guide.* Philadelphia: Lippincott Williams & Wilkins.

CONCEPT

An increased hematocrit level indicates dehydration.

POINTERS

Hematocrit is the measure of the percentage of red blood cells in the total blood volume.

Normal adult levels
Male   42% to 52%
Female   37% to 47%

Abnormal Findings

Increased levels:	Decreased levels:
Shock	**S**evere malnutrition
Polycythemia	**L**eukemia
Eclampsia	**O**rgan failure
Erythrocytosis	**W**eakness due to
Dehydration	anemia

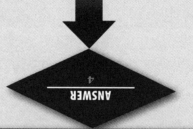

QUESTION

Which of the following blood tests is related to diabetic ketoacidosis?

1. Creatinine: 1.4 mg/dL
2. Total lipids: 100 mg/dL
3. Hemoglobin: 14 mg/dL
4. Hematocrit: 55%

ANSWER

4

RATIONALE

A hematocrit of 55% is elevated and is indicative of dehydration, which is one of the characteristics of diabetic ketoacidosis.

REFERENCE

Nettina, S. M. (2007). *The Lippincott manual of nursing practice* (8th ed., Philippine ed.). Philadelphia: Lippincott Williams & Wilkins.

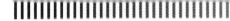
CONCEPT

For clients with heart failure, it is difficult to breathe while in supine position.

POINTERS

Discharge instructions for clients with heart failure

- PRIORITY: Physical and emotional rest
- Avoid high sodium foods
- Eat high potassium foods like apricots, bananas, and cantaloupe
- Take cardiac glycosides as prescribed and report signs of toxicity such as anorexia, vomiting, and yellowish vision
- Notify the doctor if any of the following occurs:
  ▸ Irregular pulse or pulse less than 60 bpm
  ▸ Swollen ankles
  ▸ Decreased urine output
  ▸ Weight gain of 3 to 5 lbs in a week
  ▸ Paroxysmal nocturnal dyspnea
  ▸ Dry cough
  ▸ Palpitations

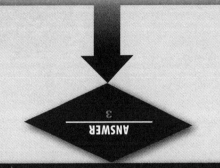

QUESTION

Which of the following questions is relevant for the nurse to ask the client with congestive heart failure?

1. "Do you urinate often?"
2. "Do you exercise regularly?"
3. "Where do you sleep at night?"
4. "How often do you move your bowels in a day?"

ANSWER

3

RATIONALE

Clients with heart failure usually sleep on a recliner to relieve paroxysmal nocturnal dyspnea.

NCLEX-RN CATEGORY Physiological Adaptation

REFERENCE

Nettina, S. M. (2007). *The Lippincott manual of nursing practice* (8th ed., Philippine ed.). Philadelphia: Lippincott Williams & Wilkins.

148

CONCEPT

Raynaud's disease is precipitated by exposure to cold and increased stress.

POINTERS

- Raynaud's disease is a vasospastic condition of arteries of the hands that occurs with exposure to cold or stress.
- Intermittent arteriolar vasoconstriction occurs.
- Allen's test reveals circulatory problems.
- Avoid cold weather.
- Wear leather gloves when getting anything from the refrigerator.
- Stop smoking.
- Administer vasodilators as ordered.

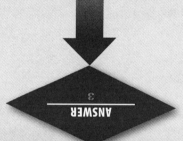

QUESTION

Which of the following discharge instructions is the priority for a client with Raynaud's disease?

1. "Wear clean latex gloves when getting anything from the refrigerator."
2. "Wear sterile gloves when getting anything from the refrigerator."
3. "Wear leather gloves when getting anything from the refrigerator."
4. "Wear rubber gloves when getting anything from the refrigerator."

ANSWER

3

RATIONALE

A client with Raynaud's disease should be instructed to wear leather gloves when getting anything from the refrigerator because vasospasm is triggered by exposure to cold temperatures.

REFERENCE

Nettina, S. M. (2007). *The Lippincott manual of nursing practice* (8th ed., Philippine ed.). Philadelphia: Lippincott Williams & Wilkins.

SUBJECT Cardiac Catheterization

CONCEPT

The distal pulse is assessed after catheterization.

POINTERS

Post-cardiac catheterization care

- Monitor the vital signs every 30 minutes for 2 hours initially.
- Notify the physician if any of the following occurs:

  Pale or cyanotic extremity

  Undetectable or sudden loss of peripheral pulse or signs of dysrhythmias

  Localized tingling

  Sensory deficits like numbness

  Extremity that is cool
- Keep the extremity extended for 4 to 6 hours.
- Maintain strict bed rest for 6 to 12 hours. Do not elevate the head of the bed more than 15 degrees.

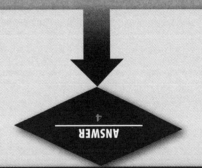

QUESTION

After femoral cardiac catheterization of a client, which of the following doctor's order should the nurse question?

1. Put the client in a supine position for 6–8 hours
2. Apply a pressure dressing at the insertion site for 24 hours
3. Check the color and pulse of the legs every hour for 4 hours
4. Check the brachial pulses every hour for 4 hours

ANSWER

4

RATIONALE

Note that the femoral vein was used for vascular access during catheterization, therefore checking the brachial pulse is not appropriate. The distal pulse in the affected leg should have been assessed.

149

NCLEX-RN CATEGORY **Reduction of Risk Potential**

REFERENCE

Pagana, K. D., & Pagana, T. J. (2006). *Mosby's diagnostic and laboratory test reference* (8th ed.). St. Louis, MO: Mosby-Year Book.

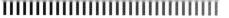

SUBJECT Viagra and Nitroglycerine

CONCEPT

Viagra and nitroglycerine can cause fatal hypotension when taken together.

POINTERS

Contraindications to Viagra

Children
Cardiac disease
Hepatic or renal dysfunction
Allergy to the drug
Women

QUESTION

Which of the following data in a client's history would contraindicate the use of sildalafil (Viagra)?

1. Angina pectoris
2. Urinary tract infection
3. Impotence
4. Slight temperature elevation

ANSWER

1

RATIONALE

Viagra and nitroglycerine should not be taken together because both drugs are vasodilators and therefore may cause severe hypotension. Nitroglycerine is usually used to manage angina pectoris.

REFERENCE
Karch, A. M. (2007). 2008 *Lippincott's nursing drug guide*. Philadelphia: Lippincott Williams & Wilkins.

CONCEPT

Atacand prevents vasoconstriction leading to decreased blood pressure.

POINTERS

Common side effects of Atacand

Rash
Abdominal pain
Nausea
Diarrhea

Report:
- Fever
- Chills
- Dizziness
- Pregnancy

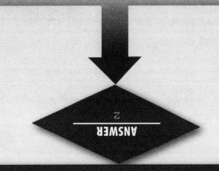

QUESTION

Candesartan cilexitil (Atacand) is usually prescribed to clients for which of the following purposes?

1. To treat diarrhea
2. To decrease blood pressure
3. To enhance glucose utilization
4. To decrease ammonia absorption

ANSWER

2

RATIONALE

Atacand is given to a client with hypertension because it decreases high blood pressure.

REFERENCE

Karch, A. M. (2007). *2008 Lippincott's nursing drug guide.* Philadelphia: Lippincott Williams & Wilkins.

CONCEPT

Distal peripheral pulses should be assessed after cardiac catheterization.

POINTERS

- Cardiac catheterization measures oxygen concentration, saturation, tension, and pressure in various chambers of the heart. It determines the need for cardiac surgery.
- Obtain informed consent.
- Assess for allergy.
- NPO for 6 hours before the procedure
- After procedure: check peripheral and apical pulses every 15 minutes for 2–4 hours. Check puncture site for bleeding. Keep a 20 lb sandbag at the bedside to apply pressure in case bleeding occurs.
- Keep extremity extended for 4–6 hours.
- Notify the physician if the client complains of numbness, tingling, cool extremities, is pale or cyanotic, or if there is sudden loss of peripheral pulses.

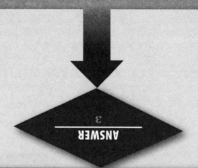

QUESTION

After cardiac catheterization, the client complains of a sudden loss of peripheral pulses. What should the nurse do?

1. Document the findings in the chart
2. Inform the client that it is an expected effect after the procedure
3. Report the findings to the physician immediately
4. Apply a 20 lb sandbag at the distal portion of the extremities

ANSWER

3

RATIONALE

After cardiac catheterization, the nurse should notify the physician of the manifestations of circulatory and nerve impairment such as numbness, tingling, cool extremities, pallor or cyanosis, or a sudden loss of peripheral pulses.

REFERENCE

Nettina, S. M. (2007). *The Lippincott manual of nursing practice* (8th ed., Philippine ed.). Philadelphia: Lippincott Williams & Wilkins.

CONCEPT

ATSO$_4$ is used in complete heart block where the ECG reveals prolonged PR interval (more than 0.20 seconds).

POINTERS

- Complete heart block is due to an altered transmission of wave impulses from the SA node to the AV node.
- ECG reveals prolonged PR interval.
- Monitor the client's ECG.
- Prepare the client for pacemaker insertion.
- A common sign of pacemaker failure is hiccups.
- Atropine sulfate is given as a vagolytic.

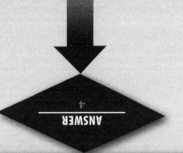

QUESTION

The ECG of a client reveals a PR interval of .32 seconds. Which of the following drugs should the nurse anticipate that the doctor will order?

1. Aspirin
2. Enoxaparin sodium (Lovenox)
3. Deferoxamine mesylate (Desferal)
4. Atropine sulfate

ANSWER

4

RATIONALE

An ECG tracing with a PR interval of 0.32 seconds is indicative of complete heart block, hence the nurse should anticipate that the doctor will order atropine SO$_4$, an anticholinergic drug, to increase the heart rate.

REFERENCE

Nettina, S. M. (2007). *The Lippincott manual of nursing practice* (8th ed., Philippine ed.). Philadelphia: Lippincott Williams & Wilkins.

153

NCLEX-RN CATEGORY Physiological Adaptation

154

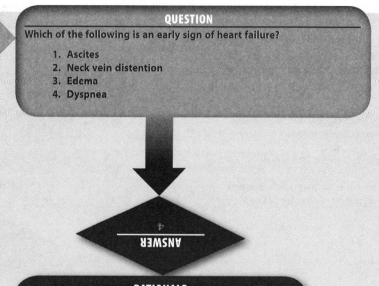

CONCEPT

Left-sided heart failure develops before right-sided heart failure.

POINTERS

- Manifestations of left-sided heart failure include:
  - ‣ Dyspnea on exertion
  - ‣ Orthopnea
  - ‣ Fatigue
  - ‣ Cough
  - ‣ Crackles

- Manifestations of right-sided heart failure include:
  - ‣ Jugular vein distention
  - ‣ Ascites
  - ‣ Peripheral edema
  - ‣ Hepatomegaly

QUESTION

Which of the following is an early sign of heart failure?

1. Ascites
2. Neck vein distention
3. Edema
4. Dyspnea

ANSWER

4

RATIONALE

Dyspnea is the earliest sign of left-sided heart failure.

REFERENCE

Nettina, S. M. (2007). *The Lippincott manual of nursing practice* (8th ed., Philippine ed.). Philadelphia: Lippincott Williams & Wilkins.

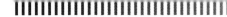

CONCEPT

A normal urine output indicates adequate fluid circulation in the body.

POINTERS

- Cardiogenic shock is due to the heart's inability to pump an adequate amount of blood.
- Early warning signs include altered consciousness, tachycardia, and tachypnea.

PRIORITY: Assess the client's circulatory status (palpate the radial pulse first)

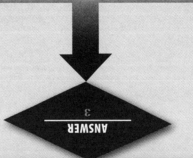

QUESTION

Which of the following assessment findings best indicates a positive reponse to the treatment of cardiogenic shock?

1. Normal cardiac rhythm
2. Normal blood pressure
3. Urine output of 60 ml in 2 hours
4. Respiratory rate of 16 breaths per minute

ANSWER

3

RATIONALE

A urine output of 60 ml in 2 hours is indicative of adequate fluid circulation. The normal urine output is 30 to 60 ml/hour.

REFERENCE

Nettina, S. M. (2007). *The Lippincott manual of nursing practice* (8th ed., Philippine ed.). Philadelphia: Lippincott Williams & Wilkins.

SUBJECT Congenital Heart Disease (CHD)

CONCEPT

Brow sweating during feeding may suggest the presence of congenital heart disease in infants.

POINTERS

Common manifestations of infants with CHD

- Weak sucking
- Turns blue with feeding
- Takes an overly long time to feed
- Brow sweating during feeding

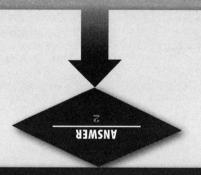

QUESTION

Which of the following observations in a neonate requires further investigation by the nurse?

1. Occasional respiratory infection
2. Falling asleep after a few minutes of feeding
3. Rapid growth
4. Acrocyanosis

ANSWER

2

RATIONALE

Falling asleep after a few minutes of feeding indicates weak sucking and easy fatigability found in infants with congenital heart disease.

REFERENCE

Nettina, S. M. (2007). *The Lippincott manual of nursing practice* (8th ed., Philippine ed.). Philadelphia: Lippincott Williams & Wilkins.

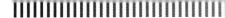

CONCEPT

Bed rest is indicated for clients with inflammatory conditions of the heart.

POINTERS

- Pericarditis is the inflammation of the pericardium.
- Sharp pain that radiates to the neck, shoulders, back, and arms is a common manifestation.
- Pleuritic chest pain increases with deep inspiration and decreases when the client sits up and leans forward.

PRIORITY: Bed rest

QUESTION

Which of the following interventions is not appropriate for a client with pericarditis?

1. Complete bed rest
2. Ambulate the client for 30 minutes daily
3. Semi-Fowler's position
4. Low sodium diet

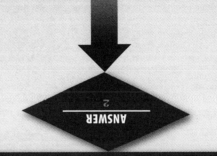

ANSWER

2

RATIONALE

Clients with pericarditis should remain on bed rest when chest pain, fever and friction rub occur.

REFERENCE

Nettina, S. M. (2007). *The Lippincott manual of nursing practice* (8th ed., Philippine ed.). Philadelphia: Lippincott Williams & Wilkins.

CONCEPT

Diuretics promote excretion of excess fluids.

POINTERS

- Myocardial infarction is the destruction of cardiac tissue due to reduced coronary blood flow.
- There is lower sternal pain characterized as crushing or excruciating that is not relieved by rest and nitroglycerine.
- The following substances elevate in the following order: myoglobin, troponin, creatinine phosphokinase, and lactic dehydrogenase.
- ECG reveals ST segment elevation or depression and T wave inversion.
- PRIORITY: Administer oxygen
- Position the client in semi-Fowler's position.
- Administer demerol to relieve the pain.
- Maintain a low fat, low cholesterol, low sodium diet.

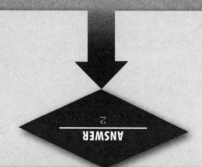

QUESTION

A client with myocardial infarction develops rales in both lung fields. Which of the following doctor's orders should the nurse carry out first?

1. Measure abdominal circumference
2. Furosemide (Lasix) 40 mg intravenously STAT
3. Obtain serum potassium level
4. Monitor urine output

ANSWER

2

RATIONALE

Rales heard in both lung fields in a client with MI is indicative of congestion. Diuretics such as furosemide should be administered to promote excretion of excess fluids from the lungs.

REFERENCE

Nettina, S. M. (2007). The Lippincott manual of nursing practice (8th ed., Philippine ed.). Philadelphia: Lippincott Williams & Wilkins.

CONCEPT

Legionnaire's disease is common among elderly chronically ill clients with long hospitalizations.

POINTERS

- Legionnaire's disease is an acute bronchopneumonia probably transmitted by an airborne route.
- Erythromycin is the drug of choice.
- Assess the client for signs of shock (decreased blood pressure, thready pulse, diaphoresis, and clammy skin).

QUESTION

Which of the following clients is least at risk for Legionnaire's disease?

1. A client with chronic renal failure
2. A client with diabetes mellitus
3. A newly admitted client with edema
4. An elderly client hospitalized for chronic obstructive pulmonary disease

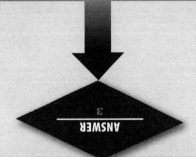

ANSWER 3

RATIONALE

Legionnaire's disease most likely affects: middle-aged, immuno-compromised clients and clients with chronic underlying disease such as diabetes, chronic renal failure, or chronic obstructive pulmonary disease.

REFERENCE

Springhouse (Ed.). (2000). *Handbook of infectious diseases.* Philadelphia: Lippincott Williams, & Wilkins.

159

NCLEX-RN CATEGORY **Physiological Adaptation**

CONCEPT

Multi-drug therapy prevents development of a resistant TB organism.

POINTERS

Multi-drug therapy

Rifampicin → causes:
- Red-orange discoloration of body secretions
- Nausea
- Vomiting

INH → causes:
- Peripheral neuritis

3H epatitis
epatic enzyme elevation
ypersensitivity

Ethambutol → causes:
- Optic neuritis (diminished red-green color discrimination)

QUESTION

What is the purpose of the combination drug therapy for a client with tuberculosis (TB)?

1. To prolong the effects of the drug.
2. To decrease the side effects of the drugs.
3. To decrease the duration of the treatment.
4. To prevent the development of resistant strains of the TB organism.

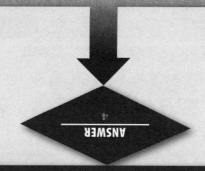

ANSWER

4

RATIONALE

Multi-drug therapy for tuberculosis is required to prevent development of drug resistant strains of the TB organism.

REFERENCE

Springhouse (Ed.). (2000). *Handbook of infectious diseases.* Philadelphia: Lippincott Williams, & Wilkins.

SUBJECT Mantoux Test (PPD skin test)

CONCEPT

A Mantoux test does not differentiate previous and present exposure to mycobacterium tuberculosis.

POINTERS

Interpretation of Mantoux test result

- Normal findings: Negative reaction (less than 5 mm skin induration)
- The area of redness around the skin induration (hardening) is not included when measuring the induration.
- 5 mm or more induration is considered positive for people with:
  - ▶ Known HIV or unknown HIV but with risk factors for HIV
  - ▶ Recent contact with active tuberculosis
  - ▶ Fibrotic changes on chest X-ray consistent with healed TB
- 10 mm or more induration is considered positive in people with:
  - ▶ Medical conditions like diabetes mellitus, end stage renal disease, prolonged corticosteroid therapy
  - ▶ Origin from areas of the world where TB is common (Asia, Latin America, Africa)
  - ▶ Children under 4 years old
- The test result is read in 48 to 72 hours.
- Report positive tests to the physician immediately.

QUESTION

Which of the following questions should the nurse ask the client before a Mantoux test is done?

1. "Do you have a family history of TB?"
2. "Did you have a positive test for TB in the past?"
3. "Do you have friends who have been treated for TB?"
4. "Do you have any allergies?"

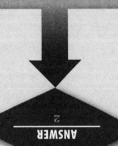

ANSWER

2

RATIONALE

Tuberculin skin test (PPD) or Mantoux test is used to detect tuberculosis exposure, either past or present, active or inactive. Hence, it is appropriate for the nurse to obtain history of exposure to tuberculosis before the test is done.

REFERENCE

Nettina, S. M. (2007). *The Lippincott manual of nursing practice* (8th ed., Philippine ed.). Philadelphia: Lippincott Williams & Wilkins.

SUBJECT Isoniazid (INH)

CONCEPT

INH causes hepatotoxicity.

POINTERS

- INH is an antituberculous agent.
- It is best taken on an empty stomach.
- Report tingling sensations in the lower extremities to the physician; they indicate peripheral neuropathy.
- Avoid alcohol.
- Liver function studies should be done before the start of therapy.
- Therapeutic effects generally occur in 2–3 weeks.
- Administer with vitamin B$_6$ to prevent peripheral neuropathy.

NCLEX-RN CATEGORY Pharmacological and Parenteral Therapies

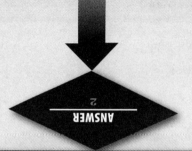

QUESTION

In a client receiving isoniazid (INH), which of the following laboratory data needs to be reported to the physician?

1. Urine output of 30 ml/hr
2. Elevated AST and ALT
3. Serum potassium level of 3.7 mEq/L
4. Decreased blood pressure

ANSWER

2

RATIONALE

Elevated AST and ALT levels are indicative of drug-induced hepatitis, a common side effect of isoniazid.

REFERENCE

Karch, A. M. (2007). *2008 Lippincott's nursing drug guide.* Philadelphia: Lippincott Williams & Wilkins.

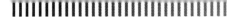

SUBJECT Tuberculosis

CONCEPT

Immunosupressed clients are at risk for TB.

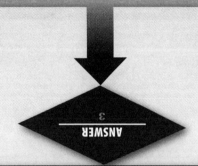

QUESTION

Which of the following clients is most at risk for tuberculosis?

1. A 12-year-old child with asthma
2. A 45-year-old obese client
3. A 68-year-old client who is taking prednisone
4. A 20-year-old pregnant client with leg edema

ANSWER

3

RATIONALE

Prednisone is a steroid that decreases immune resistance to infection, making the client at risk of becoming infected with tuberculosis.

POINTERS

- TB is a respiratory infection caused by mycobacterium tuberculosis. Risk factors for infection reactivation include gastrectomy, Hodgkins' disease, leukemia, Silicosis, AIDS, and use of steroids.
- Instruct the client to cover the mouth and nose when coughing. Implement airborne precautions.
- A combination of drugs is used to prevent bacterial resistance. It should be taken for 6–12 months. Drugs include rifampicin, INH, streptomycin, and ethambutol.
- Noncompliance can lead to drug-resistant TB. Treatment for this may require administration of a second line of drugs such as capreomycin, streptomycin, para-aminosalicylic acid, cycloserine, amikacin, and quinolone drugs.

163

NCLEX-RN CATEGORY **Physiological Adaptation**

REFERENCE

Springhouse (Ed.). (2000). *Handbook of infectious diseases.* Philadelphia: Lippincott Williams & Wilkins.

CONCEPT

The priority in carbon monoxide poisoning is to assess airway and breathing.

POINTERS

- The normal carboxyhemoglobin level is less than 12%.
- Severe carbon monoxide poisoning is present at levels greater than 30%.
- Reverse hypoxia by administering 100% oxygen.

QUESTION

Which of the following interventions is the priority in carbon monoxide poisoning?

1. Administer 100% oxygen
2. Assess the airway
3. Obtain arterial blood gas levels
4. Monitor the vital signs

ANSWER

2

RATIONALE

Assessing for patent airway and spontaneous breathing are priority interventions in a client with carbon monoxide poisoning.

REFERENCE

Nettina, S. M. (2007). *The Lippincott manual of nursing practice* (8th ed., Philippine ed.). Philadelphia: Lippincott Williams & Wilkins.

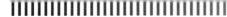

CONCEPT

The normal oxygen saturation is 95–98%.

POINTERS

- Oxygen saturation is an important index of tissue perfusion and calculation of oxygen delivery.
- Oximetry is a method of monitoring arterial blood oxygen saturation.
- Oximetry can be used to assess the body's response to drugs like theophylline.

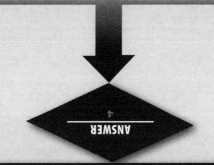

QUESTION

After a motor vehicular accident, which of the following findings should a nurse give priority in planning for the care of a client with a chest injury?

1. Heart rate of 65 beats per minute and respiratory rate of 22 breaths per minute
2. Body temperature of 37.1°C
3. Arterial carbon dioxide level of 38 mm Hg and carboxyhemoglobin level of 2%
4. Oxygen saturation of 83%

ANSWER

4

RATIONALE

An oxygen saturation of less than 88% is indicative of hypoxia, which requires immediate intervention.

REFERENCE

Nettina, S. M. (2007). *The Lippincott manual of nursing practice* (8th ed., Philippine ed.). Philadelphia: Lippincott Williams & Wilkins.

NCLEX-RN CATEGORY Reduction of Risk Potential

CONCEPT

Rest periods should be provided in between the activities of a client with asthma.

POINTERS

- Asthma is due to abnormal bronchial hyperactivity to certain substances.
- Dyspnea is a common sign.
- ABG reveals respiratory acidosis.
- Instruct the client to avoid the 3Es: exercise (especially in cold weather), environmental factors (like dust or pollen), and emotional factors.
- Instruct the client to sit upright and lean forward on a table during asthmatic attacks.
- Encourage the client to do pursed-lip breathing.

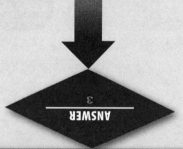

QUESTION

Which of the following activities is appropriate for a 12-year-old child with asthma?

1. Soccer
2. 1,500 meter run
3. Baseball
4. Long distance biking

ANSWER

3

RATIONALE

Baseball is an appropriate activity for an asthmatic child because it allows for rest periods during the game.

REFERENCE

Nettina, S. M. (2007). *The Lippincott manual of nursing practice* (8th ed., Philippine ed.). Philadelphia: Lippincott Williams & Wilkins.

SUBJECT ASA (Aspirin)

CONCEPT

Aspirin causes bronchospasm.

POINTERS

- Aspirin is an anti-inflammatory, anti-pyretic, analgesic, anti-platelet aggregate.
- Best taken on full stomach
- Tinnitus indicates toxicity.
- Avoid other over-the-counter cold remedies.
- May cause bronchospasm
- Assess the client for bleeding tendencies.
- Induce vomiting if overdose occurs.

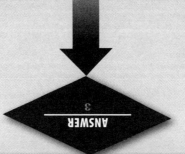

QUESTION

A client who is newly diagnosed with asthma comes to the clinic for evaluation. The nurse needs to notify the doctor when the client says:

1. "I have difficulty breathing at night."
2. "I make sure that I attend my baseball practice."
3. "I have been diagnosed with juvenile rheumatoid arthritis."
4. "I know this condition may affect my activities."

ANSWER

3

RATIONALE

Aspirin, a drug given to clients with rheumatoid arthritis, is contraindicated in clients with asthma because it causes bronchospasm.

167

REFERENCE

Karch, A. M. (2007). *2008 Lippincott's nursing drug guide*. Philadelphia: Lippincott Williams & Wilkins.

NCLEX-RN CATEGORY Pharmacological and Parenteral Therapies

CONCEPT

Propranolol causes bronchospasm.

POINTERS

- Propanolol Is an antIanginal, antiarrythmic, antihypertensive; it reduces portal pressure and decreases the risk of bleeding from esophageal varices.
- Best taken with meals
- Avoid driving; do not discontinue abruptly
- Check the BP; it may cause hypotension
- May cause bronchospasm

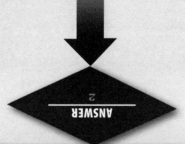

QUESTION

A 30-year-old client is receiving theophylline. Which of the following drugs is contraindicated?

1. Epinephrine
2. Propanolol (Inderal)
3. Enoxacin (Penetrex)
4. Dexamethasone (Decadron)

ANSWER

2

RATIONALE

A client receiving theophylline is considered as being treated for asthma. Propanolol is a beta-blocker and a common side effect is bronchospasm. Therefore, propanolol should not be given to a client who is being treated for asthma.

REFERENCE
Gapuz, R. *The ABCs of passing foreign nursing exams.* Philippines: Gapuz Publications.

CONCEPT

A client with emphysema should avoid powerful odors, extremes of temperature, pets, fireplaces, and feather pillows.

QUESTION

Which of the following factors can trigger shortness of breath in a client with emphysema? Select all that apply.

1. Pet dog
2. Fireplace dust
3. Mild deodorant
4. Feather pillow
5. Moderate room temperature

POINTERS

- Emphysema is due to the destruction of alveoli, narrowing of small airways, and the trapping of air resulting in loss of lung elasticity.
- Barrel chest (increase in the anteroposterior diameter of the chest) is a late sign.
- ABG reveals respiratory acidosis.
- Keep the client in a sitting-up position.
- Administer low flow oxygen.
- Encourage the client to do pursed-lip breathing.
- Instruct the client to avoid powerful odors, extremes of temperature, pets, fireplaces, and feather pillows.

ANSWER

1, 2, 4

RATIONALE

A pet dog, fireplace dust, and feather pillow are among the factors that can trigger shortness of breath in a client with emphysema.

169

NCLEX-RN CATEGORY **Physiological Adaptation**

REFERENCE

Nettina, S. M. (2007). *The Lippincott manual of nursing practice* (8th ed., Philippine ed.). Philadelphia: Lippincott Williams & Wilkins.

CONCEPT

Clients with cystic fibrosis should be encouraged to perform deep breathing exercise.

POINTERS

Exercises for clients with cystic fibrosis

- Coughing
- Deep breathing
- Huffing
- Blowing

QUESTION

Which of the following instruments is best for a child with cystic fibrosis who wants to join the school band?

1. Piano
2. Drums
3. Lyre
4. Trumpet

ANSWER

4

RATIONALE

A client with cystic fibrosis is encouraged to do breathing exercises to prevent and minimize respiratory complications. Therefore, it is appropriate for a child with cystic fibrosis to use trumpet (blowing instrument) because it stimulates deep breathing.

REFERENCE

Nettina, S. M. (2007). *The Lippincott manual of nursing practice* (8th ed., Philippine ed.). Philadelphia: Lippincott Williams & Wilkins.

SUBJECT Opioids

CONCEPT
Opioids cause respiratory depression.

POINTERS
- Opioids produce analgesia.
- It may cause dizziness, drowsiness, and disorientation.
- Report any of the following to the physician:
  ▸ Severe nausea
  ▸ Vomiting
  ▸ Constipation
  ▸ Shortness of breath
  ▸ Difficulty breathing

QUESTION
Which of the following assessment parameters should the nurse monitor in a client who is receiving opioids?

1. Heart rate
2. Temperature
3. Urine output
4. Respiratory rate

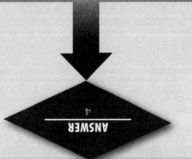

ANSWER
4

RATIONALE
The respiratory rate must be monitored closely in a client receiving opioids.

REFERENCE
Karch, A. M. (2007). *2008 Lippincott's nursing drug guide.* Philadelphia: Lippincott Williams & Wilkins.

SUBJECT Cystic Fibrosis

CONCEPT

Meconium ileus in the neonate may indicate cystic fibrosis.

POINTERS

- Cystic fibrosis is characterized by blockage of the exocrine glands (pancreas, respiratory, salivary and sweat glands) due to excessive production of viscid mucus. It is an autosomal recessive disorder. There is a 25% chance of disease transmission for every pregnancy and a 50% chance of trait transmission for every pregnancy.
- Meconium ileus is a common finding.
- Sweat chloride test reveals increased chloride levels.
- Perform postural drainage before meals and at bedtime.
- Administer pancreatic enzyme with each meal.
- Maintain high calorie, high sodium diet.
- Refer the parents of the child to a geneticist.

QUESTION

Which of the following statements made by the mother of a newborn may possibly indicate meconium ileus?

1. "My child didn't pass out his first stool until his second day."
2. "My child did not void in his first 24 hours of birth."
3. "My child had his first stool on his third day."
4. "My child's abdomen looks bloated."

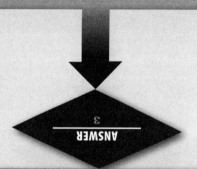

ANSWER

3

RATIONALE

Meconium ileus often occurs in infants with cystic fibrosis. It indicates that the bowel is obstructed by thick intestinal secretions. Therefore, a child having his first stool on his third day is most likely having meconium ileus.

REFERENCE

Nettina, S. M. (2007). *The Lippincott manual of nursing practice* (8th ed., Philippine ed.). Philadelphia: Lippincott Williams & Wilkins.

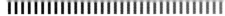

SUBJECT Ribavirin (Virazole)

CONCEPT

Ribavirin is contraindicated in pregnant and lactating clients.

POINTERS

- Virazole is an antiviral agent.
- The drug can cause cardio-respiratory arrest.
- Report the development of dizziness, confusion, and shortness of breath to the physician.
- The most frequent adverse effects related to the use of aerosolized ribavirin include headache and eye irritation.
- Contradindications include allergy to the drug, COPD, pregnancy, and lactation.

QUESTION

Which of the following visitors should the nurse restrict from visiting an infant who is on ribavirin (Virazole) due to respiratory syncytial virus (RSV)?

1. A 10-year-old neighbor
2. A hypertensive grandmother
3. A pregnant cousin
4. An aunt with a cold

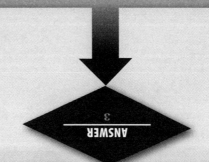

ANSWER

3

RATIONALE

A pregnant woman should keep herself from visiting a relative who is on ribavirin therapy because exposure to the drug can cause fetal damage.

173

NCLEX-RN CATEGORY Pharmacological and Parenteral Therapies

REFERENCE

Karch, A. M. (2007). *2008 Lippincott's nursing drug guide*. Philadelphia: Lippincott Williams & Wilkins.

CONCEPT

The initial intervention for a client who is choking is to establish an airway.

POINTERS

Heimlich maneuver

A. Conscious client
1. Stand behind the client and wrap your arms around the waist.
2. Make a fist with one hand and position it between the navel and the xiphoid process.
3. Grasp the fist with the other hand.
4. Make quick upward thrusts.
B. Unconscious, lying down client
1. Keep the client in flat position.
2. Face the client's head and kneel astride the client's thigh.
3. Position the heel of one hand on the client's abdomen between the navel and the xiphoid process.
4. Place the hand on top of the other and make quick upward thrusts.

QUESTION

While eating in the restaurant, the nurse hears someone yell, "Help! My cousin is choking!" The first intervention is to:

1. Give him an abdominal thrust
2. Call the doctor
3. Place him in supine position
4. Ask him "Can you talk?"

ANSWER

4

RATIONALE

Establishing a patent airway involves assessment of:

- Weak cough
- Inability to speak
- Respiratory distress
- Cyanosis
- High pitched sound on inspiration

REFERENCE

Nettina, S. M. (2007). *The Lippincott manual of nursing practice* (8th ed., Philippine ed.). Philadelphia: Lippincott Williams & Wilkins.

CONCEPT

Treatment for celiac disease involves lifetime avoidance of:

   Barley
   Rye
   Oats
   Wheat

POINTERS

- Celiac disease is characterized by a permanent inability to tolerate dietary gluten in the small intestines.
- Small bowel biopsy indicates abnormal mucosa.
- Treatment includes lifetime avoidance of:
  - **B**arley
  - **R**ye
  - **O**ats
  - **W**heat (gluten-free diet)
- Foods that are allowed include corn, cereals, soybeans, and rice. If the client attends a party, instruct the parent to prepare a homemade cake for the child to bring to the party since commercially prepared cakes are made of wheat. Refer the parents to a geneticist.

QUESTION

Which of the following foods are allowed for a client with celiac disease? Select all that apply.

1. Cereals
2. Oatmeal
3. Rice cake
4. Vanilla cake
5. Soybeans
6. Corn flakes
7. Wheat bread

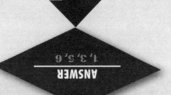

ANSWER

1, 3, 5, 6

RATIONALE

Celiac disease is a genetic disease involving malabsorption of many nutrients resulting from pathologic changes in the small intestinal mucosa induced by ingestion of gluten.

Foods that are allowed include corn, cereals, soybeans, and rice.

REFERENCE
Gapuz, R. *The ABCs of passing foreign nursing exams.* Philippines: Gapuz Publications.

CONCEPT

The normal gastric residual volume of a client is less than 50% of the total amount of tube feedings.

POINTERS

Assessing gastric residual volume

- Gastric residual volume is measured before each intermittent feeding and every 4 to 8 hours for continuous feedings.
- McClave et al. (1992) suggested that a residual volume of 200 ml or more in a client with nasogastric tubes or a residual volume of 100 ml for clients with a gastrostomy tube may indicate feeding intolerance.
  ▸ McClave, S. A., Snider, H. L., & Lowen, C. C. et al. (1992). Use of residual volume as a marker for enteral feeding intolerance: Prospective blinded comparison with physical examination and radiologic findings. *Journal of Parenteral and Enteral Nutrition, 16*(2), 99–105.

QUESTION

A client received 200 ml of tube feedings. The nurse can administer the next feeding if there is:

1. A gastric residual volume of 150 ml
2. A gastric residual volume of 80 ml
3. A gastric residual volume of 120 ml
4. A gastric residual volume of 200 ml

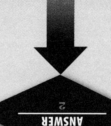

ANSWER

2

RATIONALE

A normal gastric residual volume should be less than 50% of the total amount of tube feedings. The nurse could therefore administer the next feeding when the gastric residual volume is 80 ml, which is less than 50% of 200 ml.

REFERENCE

Smeltzer, S. C., Bare, B. G., Hinkle, J. L., & Cheever, K. H. (2006). *Brunner and Suddarth's textbook of medical-surgical nursing.* Philadelphia: Lippincott Williams & Wilkins.

CONCEPT

Bolus feeding in a client with a nasogastric tube should resemble normal meal feeding.

POINTERS

- Check residual volume every 4 hours before each feeding or before giving medicine.
- The NGT is removed when bowel peristalsis returns.
- In bolus tube feeding, approximately 300 to 400 ml of formula is administered over a 30 to 60 minute period every 3 to 6 hours.

QUESTION

Bolus tube feedings are best given at which of the following times?

1. At midday in between periods of rest
2. Before the client goes to bed
3. Before the client watches his favorite late night TV show
4. In the late afternoon and at dawn

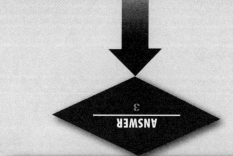

ANSWER

3

RATIONALE

Bolus feeding is best given before the client watches his favorite late night TV show because this schedule resembles a normal feeding pattern.

REFERENCE

Nettina, S. M. (2007). *The Lippincott manual of nursing practice* (8th ed., Philippine ed.). Philadelphia: Lippincott Williams & Wilkins.

177

NCLEX-RN CATEGORY **Basic Care and Comfort**

CONCEPT

Avoid stimulants in clients with GERD.

QUESTION

Which of the following foods should the nurse instruct the client with gastroesophageal reflux disease (GERD) to avoid?

1. Milk
2. Coffee
3. Vegetables
4. Wheat bread

POINTERS

- GERD is characterized by transfer of gastric contents to the esophagus.
- A barium swallow helps establish the presence of reflux.
- Provide small, frequent, thickened feedings.
- Position the client in a flat prone or head-elevated prone position. Use an upper body harness to maintain this position.
- Administer antacids as ordered.
- Avoid stimulants.
- Prepare the client for surgery to tighten lower esophageal sphincter.

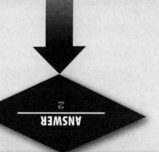

ANSWER

2

RATIONALE

Clients with GERD should avoid stimulants that reduce sphincter control (tobacco, alcohol, fatty foods, peppermint, and caffeine along with drugs like morphine, diazepam, and meperidine). Coffee contains caffeine, and should therefore be avoided.

REFERENCE

Nettina, S. M. (2007). *The Lippincott manual of nursing practice* (8th ed., Philippine ed.). Philadelphia: Lippincott Williams & Wilkins.

CONCEPT

Questran promotes excretion of bile acids in the bowels.

POINTERS

- Questran is an antihyperlipidemic agent and bile acid sequestrant.

Common side effects include:
Constipation
Abdominal cramps
Backache
Weakness and muscle pain
Exacerbation of hemorrhoids
Bleeding
Skin irritation

- Take the drug before meals.
- Mix one packet or one scoop with water, milk, juice, soup, or cereals.

QUESTION

Which of the following indicates successful use of cholestyramine (Questran) in a client with jaundice due to obstructive gallbladder disease?

1. Decreased inflammation
2. Decreased itching
3. Decreased pain
4. Decreased cholesterol levels

ANSWER

2

RATIONALE

Questran binds with bile acids that are excreted in the stools. It prevents the accumulation of bile acids on the skin, thereby decreasing itching.

REFERENCE
Karch, A. M. (2007). *2008 Lippincott's nursing drug guide.* Philadelphia: Lippincott Williams & Wilkins.

NCLEX-RN CATEGORY Pharmacological and Parenteral Therapies

CONCEPT

Clostridium difficile causes diarrhea.

POINTERS

- *Clostridium difficile* is usually associated with clindamycin use.
- It is transmitted by contaminated hands or indirectly through contaminated equipment such as bedpans, urinals, call bells, rectal thermometers, or toilet seats.
- Manifestations include foul smelling, watery, and bloody diarrhea with fever and abdominal cramps.

- PRIORITY: Place the client in a private room.

QUESTION

Which of the following oral solutions should not be given to a client with *Clostridium difficile*?

1. Pedialyte
2. Gatorade
3. Water
4. Apple juice

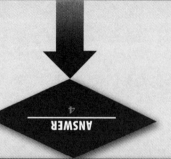

ANSWER

4

RATIONALE

Apple juice can worsen the diarrhea associated with *Clostridium difficile*.

REFERENCE

Nettina, S. M. (2007). *The Lippincott manual of nursing practice* (8th ed., Philippine ed.). Philadelphia: Lippincott Williams & Wilkins.

CONCEPT

Hepatitis A is transmitted through fecal contamination of food or water.

POINTERS

- Emphasize the importance of thorough hand washing.
- Practice standard precautions.
- Hepatitis A vaccine is recommended for children who are 12 to 23 months old. It is given in two shots at least 6 months apart as a preventive measure for hepatitis A infection.

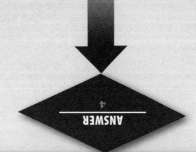

QUESTION

Hepatitis A is transmitted through:

1. Sexual intercourse
2. Contact with body secretions
3. Kissing and intimate activities
4. Contaminated food or water

ANSWER

4

RATIONALE

The mode of transmission of hepatitis A is primarily fecal-oral, usually through the ingestion of food or liquids contaminated with the virus.

REFERENCE

Nettina, S. M. (2007). *The Lippincott manual of nursing practice* (8th ed., Philippine ed.). Philadelphia: Lippincott Williams & Wilkins.

CONCEPT

Aspirin is not taken for post-operative discomfort.

QUESTION

Which of the following statements, if made by a client post liposuction, indicates a need for further instructions?

1. "I will need to drink more after surgery."
2. "I can take aspirin for my pain after the surgery."
3. "I will need to avoid jarring exercises."
4. "I will need to notify the surgeon if there is increased swelling at the site."

POINTERS

Nursing care of post-liposuction clients

- Increase fluid intake.
- Wear compression garment.
- Avoid jarring exercise.
- Report increased swelling to the surgeon.

ANSWER

2

RATIONALE

Aspirin and NSAIDs should be avoided for at least one week post surgery to prevent bleeding.

REFERENCE

Nettina, S. M. (2007). *The Lippincott manual of nursing practice* (8th ed., Philippine ed.). Philadelphia: Lippincott Williams & Wilkins.

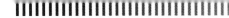
CONCEPT

Removal of ascites through abdominal paracentesis facilitates normal breathing.

POINTERS

- Abdominal paracentesis is done to examine contents of the peritoneal fluid and to relieve shortness of breath when ventilation is impaired.
- Obtain informed consent. Instruct the client to void immediately prior to the procedure to prevent accidental puncture of the bladder. During the procedure, instruct the client to sit up with feet resting on footstool. Evaluate the effect of the procedure by assessing:
  - ▶ Weight
  - ▶ Abdominal girth
  - ▶ Respiratory rate
- Notify the physician if the urine becomes bloody, pink, or red.

QUESTION

Which of the following observations indicate that abdominal paracentesis is effective?

1. Respiratory rate decreases from 36 to 20 per minute
2. Protein level decreases from 6.5 mg/dL to 5 mg/dL
3. Urine specific gravity increases from 1.016 to 1.030
4. Blood pressure decreases from 140/60 to 120/60

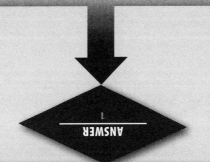

ANSWER

1

RATIONALE

Massive ascites may cause abdominal discomfort and dyspnea due to pressure exerted by the fluid against the diaphragm. A decreased respiratory rate is an indication that the client's diaphragm is able to expand.

REFERENCE

Nettina, S. M. (2007). *The Lippincott manual of nursing practice* (8th ed., Philippine ed.). Philadelphia: Lippincott Williams & Wilkins.

NCLEX-RN CATEGORY **Reduction of Risk Potential**

SUBJECT Albumin

CONCEPT

A decreased albumin level leads to edema.

POINTERS

- Fluid volume excess is also referred to as fluid overload.
- It is a condition characterized by excess of total body fluid.
- May be related to:
  - ▸ Congestive heart failure
  - ▸ Cirrhosis
  - ▸ Cushing's syndrome
- May lead to edema due to decreased albumin levels
- The normal albumin level is 3.5 to 5 mg/dL.

QUESTION

A client has an albumin level of 2.8 mg/dL. Which of the following nursing diagnoses is considered a priority?

1. Fluid volume excess
2. Fluid volume deficit
3. Altered thermoregulation
4. Fluid and electrolyte imbalance

ANSWER

1

RATIONALE

Albumin is significant in maintaining the colloid osmotic or oncotic pressure that draws water into the vasculature. Should the albumin level decrease, the oncotic pressure decreases as well, leading to movement of fluid from the vasculature to the interstitial space causing edema.

REFERENCE

Nettina, S. M. (2007). *The Lippincott manual of nursing practice* (8th ed., Philippine ed.). Philadelphia: Lippincott Williams & Wilkins.

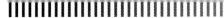

SUBJECT Hypokalemia

CONCEPT
Diuresis causes potassium excretion.

QUESTION

A client was admitted due to multiple somatic complaints. The client's laboratory results are as follows: Na 150 mEq/L; K 3.2 mEq/L; glucose 185 mg/dL; oxygen saturation of 93%. Which of the following doctor's orders should the nurse question?

1. Low sodium diet
2. Lasix in the morning
3. Blood sugar monitoring twice a day
4. Oxygen at 2–3 LPM

POINTERS

- The normal potassium level is 3.5 mEq/L to 5.0 mEq/L.
- Muscle weakness, nausea, and vomiting occur both in hypokalemia and hyperkalemia.
- Common manifestations of hypokalemia include:
  ▸ Malaise, mental confusion, muscle cramps, metabolic alkalosis
  ▸ Fatigue, flaccidity
  ▸ Depression, dysrhythmia
  ▸ Decreased GI motility
- Common manifestations of hyperkalemia
  ▸ Metabolic acidosis
  ▸ Ventricular arrhythmias
  ▸ Diarrhea

ANSWER
2

RATIONALE
Lasix, a potassium-wasting diuretic, may worsen hypokalemia.

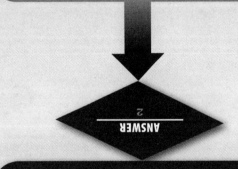

REFERENCE
Nettina, S. M. (2007). *The Lippincott manual of nursing practice* (8th ed., Philippine ed.). Philadelphia: Lippincott Williams & Wilkins.

NCLEX-RN CATEGORY **Safety and Infection Control**

CONCEPT

A high calorie, high sodium diet is indicated for a client with cystic fibrosis.

POINTERS

Diet for clients with cystic fibrosis

- Maintain a high calorie, high sodium diet.
- A pancreatic enzyme supplement should be given with all meals and snacks to facilitate fat digestion and absorption.
- Add table salt to formula or food especially during summer months to prevent hyponatremia because high concentrations of sodium occur in the client's sweat.

QUESTION

Which of the following foods is an appropriate snack for a 10-year-old child with cystic fibrosis?

1. Cookies and iced tea
2. Slices of apples and peaches
3. Toast and cheese
4. Coleslaw salad

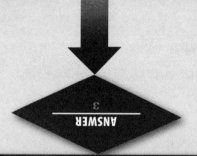

ANSWER

3

RATIONALE

A client with cystic fibrosis requires a high calorie, high sodium diet. Therefore, it is appropriate to give the child toast and cheese.

REFERENCE

Dudek, S. G. (2006). *Nutrition essentials for nursing practice* (5th ed.). Philadelphia: Lippincott Williams & Wilkins.

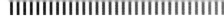

CONCEPT

Vegetarians do not eat any animal product.

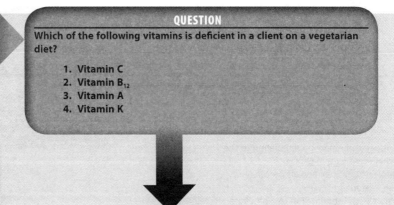

QUESTION

Which of the following vitamins is deficient in a client on a vegetarian diet?

1. Vitamin C
2. Vitamin B$_{12}$
3. Vitamin A
4. Vitamin K

POINTERS

- Seventh-Day Adventists and some Hindus are vegetarian.
- Vegetables are rich in vitamin B$_9$ (folacin) but deficient in vitamin B$_{12}$ (cyanocobalamin).

ANSWER

2

RATIONALE

Animal products are rich in vitamin B$_{12}$ and plants are generally not, therefore vegetarians have potential for vitamin B$_{12}$ deficiency because they do not eat any animal product.

REFERENCE

Springhouse (Ed.). (2005). *Nursing herbal medicine handbook*. Philadelphia: Lippincott Williams & Wilkins

NCLEX-RN CATEGORY **Basic Care and Comfort**

CONCEPT

Jaundice is usually noted first in the sclera.

POINTERS

- Cholelithiasis involves the presence of stones in the gallbladder.
- Right upper abdominal pain radiating to the right shoulder blade may occur.
- Oral cholecystography reveals presence of calcium in stones.
- Maintain a high protein, high carbohydrate, low fat diet. Assess the client for allergy to iodine, shellfish, and seafoods, since the dye used in cholecystography is iodine-based.

QUESTION

Which of the following questions should the nurse ask a client with cholelithiasis?

1. "How long ago did you notice the whites of your eyes turn yellow?"
2. "Did you notice any change in the color of your tongue?"
3. "Did you notice flapping of your hands?"
4. "Did you experience pain in your left arm?"

ANSWER

1

RATIONALE

Jaundice or icterus is a yellowish discoloration of tissues resulting from a deposit of bilirubin. A slight increase in serum bilirubin, at least 3.0 mg/dL, is best detected by examining the sclerae, which has a particularly high affinity for bilirubin due to their high elastin content.

REFERENCE

Nettina, S. M. (2007). *The Lippincott manual of nursing practice* (8th ed., Philippine ed.). Philadelphia: Lippincott Williams & Wilkins.

CONCEPT

Bloody mucoid diarrhea occurs 10–20 times in a client with ulcerative colitis, 3–4 times in a client with Crohn's disease, and it alternates with constipation in a client with diverticulitis.

POINTERS

Ulcerative colitis
- Ulceration of the mucosa of the lower colon and rectum

Crohn's disease
- Chronic inflammatory disease of the small intestines

Diverticulitis
- Inflammation of a pouch or saccular dilatation in the colon (diverticula)

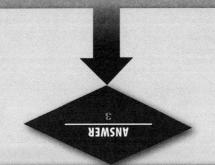

QUESTION

Which assessment finding differentiates ulcerative colitis from Crohn's disease?

1. Rapid weight loss occurs
2. Ulcerative colitis is characterized by bloody mucoid diarrhea alternating with constipation
3. The client has more frequent loose stools
4. The client is an elderly female

ANSWER

3

RATIONALE

A client who complains of more frequent loose stools suffers from ulcerative colitis rather than Crohn's disease because diarrhea occurs 10–20 times per day in ulcerative colitis.

189

REFERENCE

Nettina, S. M. (2007). *The Lippincott manual of nursing practice* (8th ed., Philippine ed.). Philadelphia: Lippincott Williams & Wilkins.

NCLEX-RN CATEGORY **Physiological Adaptation**

CONCEPT

A low fiber diet is indicated for diverticulitis. A high fiber diet is indicated for diverticulosis.

POINTERS

- In diverticulitis there is inflammation of a pouch or saccular dilatation in the colon (diverticula).
- Left lower quadrant pain occurs.
- Sigmoidoscopy confirms the diagnosis.
- Provide a low fiber diet (avoid vegetables) in diverticulitis and a high fiber diet in diverticulosis.
- Administer psyllium (Metamucil) as ordered.
- Administer meperidine (Demerol) for the relief of pain.

QUESTION

Which of the following statements made by a client with diverticulitis reflects a need for further instruction from the nurse?

1. "I need to report if a board-like abdomen develops."
2. "I eat a green salad everyday."
3. "I don't eat tomatoes."
4. "I need to take medications for pain relief."

ANSWER

2

RATIONALE

Intake of a high fiber diet in diverticulitis will increase the bulk of the stool. Residue with bacteria formation may form a hard mass (fecalith), which will compromise the blood supply and further aggravate the inflammatory process.

REFERENCE

Springhouse (Ed.). (2002). *Illustrated manual of nursing practice* (3rd ed.). Philadelphia: Lippincott Williams & Wilkins.

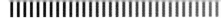

CONCEPT

Ulcerative colitis is a disorder characterized by familial predisposition.

POINTERS

- Ulcerative colitis is characterized by ulceration of the mucosa of the lower colon and rectum.
- Bloody mucoid diarrhea occurs.
- Barium enema reveals lesions.
- Avoid dairy products.
- Maintain a low residue, high protein diet.
- Avoid cold fluids.
- Teach the client's family about familial predisposition to the disease.

QUESTION

Which of the following statements made by a client indicates an understanding of ulcerative colitis?

1. "I'm glad the disease transmission ended with my father's death."
2. "The disease won't affect any member of my family."
3. "I will avoid getting in contact with fecal contaminated equipment so I won't have the disease."
4. "I am not surprised I have it because my father had the same disease."

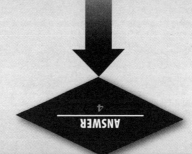

ANSWER

4

RATIONALE

Ulcerative colitis has a genetic predisposition. Therefore, the statement "I am not surprised I have it because my father had the same disease" indicates that the client is aware of his condition's causative factor.

REFERENCE

Nettina, S. M. (2007). *The Lippincott manual of nursing practice* (8th ed., Philippine ed.). Philadelphia: Lippincott Williams & Wilkins.

CONCEPT

Steroid therapy increases the risk for osteoporosis.

QUESTION

Which of the following assessment findings in a client on prolonged steroid therapy indicates a complication?

1. Weight gain
2. Easy fatigability
3. A progressive decrease in height
4. Anorexia

POINTERS

Client teaching tips on steroid therapy

- Report signs of infection like fever, redness, swelling, sore throat, and delayed wound healing.
- Report mood swings, bone pain, easy bruising, and signs of bleeding, like tarry stools.
- Long-term steroid therapy may cause osteoporosis.
- Visual disturbances may be indicative of cataracts or glaucoma.
- To minimize gastric irritation, limit the intake of alcohol, caffeine, and aspirin.
- Do not discontinue taking the drug abruptly as it may cause an adrenal crisis.

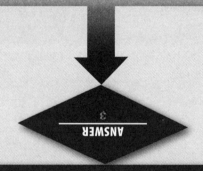

ANSWER 3

RATIONALE

Steroid therapy increases the risk for osteoporosis, manifested by a progressive decrease in height.

REFERENCE

Blicharz, M. E., Talbot, E. A., & Willens, J. S. (1994). *NSNA pharmacology*. Clinton Park, NY: Delmar.

CONCEPT

Food in the stomach decreases the absorption of Xeloda.

POINTERS

Common drugs that are best given before meals:

Bactrim
Atropine
Dalmane

Valium
Insulin
Mestinon

QUESTION

A 50-year-old with breast cancer was started on capecitabine (Xeloda). The nurse notes that the most appropriate time to administer the drug is:

1. After meals
2. Before meals
3. Without regard to meals
4. As often as the client wants to

ANSWER

2

RATIONALE

Xeloda should be taken on an empty stomach because food in the stomach decreases its absorption.

REFERENCE

Karch, A. M. (2007). *2008 Lippincott's nursing drug guide*. Philadelphia: Lippincott Williams & Wilkins.

NCLEX-RN CATEGORY **Pharmacological and Parenteral Therapies**

CONCEPT

Questran lowers low-density lipoprotein levels.

POINTERS

- Questran is an antihyperlipidemic agent and bile acid sequestrant.

Common side effects include:
Constipation
Abdominal cramps
Backache
Weakness and muscle pain
Exacerbation of hemorrhoids
Bleeding
Skin irritation

- Take the drug before meals.
- Mix one packet or one scoop with water, milk, juice, soup, or cereals.

QUESTION

Which of the following is an expected outcome for a client receiving cholestyramine (Questran)?

1. Decreased blood pressure
2. Decreased urine output
3. Decreased serum cholesterol
4. Decreased respiratory rate

ANSWER

3

RATIONALE

Cholestyramine is an antihyperlipidemic agent. Therefore an expected outcome is a decreased serum cholesterol level.

REFERENCE
Karch, A. M. (2007). *2008 Lippincott's nursing drug guide.* Philadelphia: Lippincott Williams & Wilkins.

SUBJECT Tube Drainage

CONCEPT

Absence of drainage in a tube needs to be assessed.

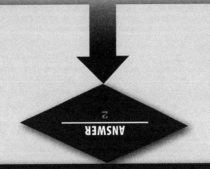

QUESTION

Which of the following clients should the nurse visit first?

1. A client with a urinary catheter drainage of 60 ml in 2 hours
2. A client with no drainage from a nephrostomy tube
3. A client with 300 ml of yellowish drainage from a T-tube
4. A client with 20 ml of bright red gastric drainage 10 hours post gastrectomy

ANSWER 2

RATIONALE

A nephrostomy tube without output requires immediate assessment and intervention because it is indicative of an obstruction.

POINTERS

T-tube
- Sudden increase in drainage (> 500 ml/24 hours) indicates obstruction.

Sengstaken-Blakemore tube
- Increased bloody drainage indicates persistent bleeding

Urinary catheter
- The normal urine output is 30 to 60 ml per hour.

Nephrostomy tube
- Urine output of less than 30 ml per hour or absence of output for more than 15 minutes should be reported to the physician.

Gastric tube
- Bright red gastric drainage is expected within 12 hours after gastrectomy.

REFERENCE

Nettina, S. M. (2007). *The Lippincott manual of nursing practice* (8th ed., Philippine ed.). Philadelphia: Lippincott Williams & Wilkins.

NCLEX-RN CATEGORY Reduction of Risk Potential

CONCEPT

Alport's syndrome is responsible for about 15% of hematuria cases in children.

POINTERS

- Alport's syndrome is more common in males.
- Diagnostic confirmation is done through a biopsy of the kidney.
- Manifestations include a slow development of deafness, clear vision, high blood pressure, and swelling of the eyes, especially in the morning.
- A low-protein diet is recommended.

QUESTION

Which of the following assessment findings is typical in a client with Alport's syndrome?

1. Nocturia
2. Cola-colored urine
3. Polyuria
4. Anuria

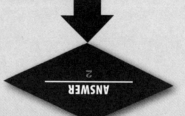

ANSWER

2

RATIONALE

Alport's syndrome is a progressive chronic glomerular nephritis inherited as an autosomal dominant disorder. A client with Alport's syndrome usually presents with hematuria or dark, smokey, cola-colored or red brown urine.

REFERENCE

Nettina, S. M. (2007). *The Lippincott manual of nursing practice* (8th ed., Philippine ed.). Philadelphia: Lippincott Williams & Wilkins.

CONCEPT

Drugs that are both nephrotoxic should not be combined.

POINTERS

Drugs that are nephrotoxic

1. Aminoglycosides (gentamicin, streptomycin, neomycin)
2. Chemotherapeutic agents (cisplatin, doxorubicin, Adriamycin)

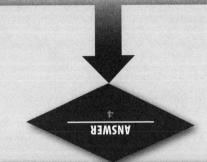

QUESTION

A client who is undergoing chemotherapy with cisplatin (Platinol) has the following doctor's orders. Which one should the nurse question?

1. Increase fluid intake
2. Arrange for BUN and creatinine tests before therapy
3. Monitor input and output
4. Administer gentamicin (Garamycin) for secondary infection

ANSWER

4

RATIONALE

Cisplatin, an antineoplastic agent, and gentamicin, an aminoglycoside antibiotic, are both nephrotoxic drugs and will further impair renal function if given in combination.

REFERENCE

Karch, A. M. (2007). *2008 Lippincott's nursing drug guide.* Philadelphia: Lippincott Williams & Wilkins.

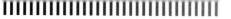
CONCEPT

Small amounts of voiding may be a sign of an overdistended bladder.

POINTERS

- Urinary retention can lead to urinary infection and possibly renal failure.
- Catheterization is done only when all other measures are unsuccessful.
- Sitz baths or warm compresses are used to relax the urinary sphincters.

QUESTION

A post-op client has 20–30 ml of urine every 15 to 30 minutes. What should the nurse do initially?

1. Apply a cold compress on the lower abdomen
2. Administer bethanecol (Mecholine) as prescribed
3. Catheterize the client
4. Palpate the bladder

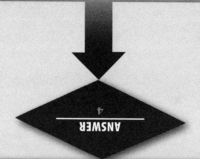

ANSWER

4

RATIONALE

A client with 20–30 ml of urine output every 15–30 minutes may be having urinary retention. The nurse should initially assess the client by palpating the bladder.

REFERENCE

Nettina, S. M. (2007). *The Lippincott manual of nursing practice* (8th ed., Philippine ed.). Philadelphia: Lippincott Williams & Wilkins.

SUBJECT Triamterene (Dyrenium)

CONCEPT

Potassium is primarily excreted in the urine.

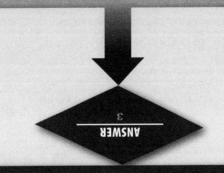

QUESTION

A client has a potassium level of 2.8 mEq/L. Which of the following doctor's orders is appropriate?

1. Chlorothiazide (Diuril)
2. Furosemide (Lasix)
3. Triamterene (Dyrenium)
4. Mannitol (Osmitrol)

ANSWER

3

RATIONALE

Triamterene is a potassium-sparing diuretic and will not worsen hypokalemia.

POINTERS

- Dyrenium is a potassium-sparing diuretic.
- It is contraindicated in hyperkalemia.
- Report any of the following to the physician:
  ‣ Change in weight of more than 3 lbs in 1 day
  ‣ Swelling of the ankles or fingers
  ‣ Fever
  ‣ Sore throat
  ‣ Unusual bleeding

REFERENCE

Karch, A. M. (2007). *2008 Lippincott's nursing drug guide.* Philadelphia: Lippincott Williams & Wilkins.

NCLEX-RN CATEGORY **Pharmacological and Parenteral Therapies**

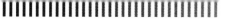

SUBJECT Chlorothiazide (Diuril)

CONCEPT
Diuril is best given in the morning.

QUESTION
Diuril is best taken at which of the following times?

1. Before breakfast
2. In the morning with meals
3. In the late afternoon
4. Before dinner

POINTERS
- Administer Diuril with food or milk.
- Record the weight.
- Common side effects:
  Steven-Johnson's syndrome
  Thrombocytopenia
  Anaphylaxis
  Renal failure

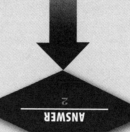

ANSWER
2

RATIONALE
Diuril causes diuresis, which may potentially disturb sleep at night. It is therefore best given in the morning and the nurse should instruct the client to stay near the bathroom.

REFERENCE
Karch, A. M. (2007). *2008 Lippincott's nursing drug guide.* Philadelphia: Lippincott Williams & Wilkins.

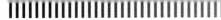

SUBJECT Furosemide (Lasix)

CONCEPT

Lasix promotes excretion of excess fluids.

POINTERS

- Lasix is a diuretic.
- It increases urine output.
- It is best given in the morning.
- Eat bananas and citrus fruits because they are good sources of potassium.
- Monitor serum potassium levels, as Lasix can cause hypokalemia.

QUESTION

Which of the following statements made by a client with ascites indicates the effectiveness of furosemide (Lasix)?

1. "I've gained much weight in a week."
2. "I can button my pants again."
3. "I still feel short of breath."
4. "I am sleeping on a recliner at night."

ANSWER

2

RATIONALE

"I can button my pants again" is indicative of decreased abdominal girth, a favorable response in a client taking furosemide.

REFERENCE

Karch, A. M. (2007). *2008 Lippincott's nursing drug guide*. Philadelphia: Lippincott Williams & Wilkins.

NCLEX-RN CATEGORY **Pharmacological and Parenteral Therapies**

SUBJECT Testicular Torsion

CONCEPT

Scrotal pain indicates testicular torsion or twisting of the spermatic cord, which is a medical emergency.

POINTERS

- Testicular torsion is the abnormal twisting of the spermatic cord.
- Common between ages 12 and 18
- Excruciating pain is the most common assessment finding.
- PRIORITY: Prepare the client for surgery.

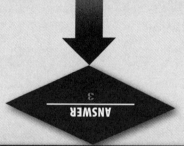

QUESTION

Which of the following clients should the nurse assess first?

1. A 40-year-old client complaining of unequal testicles
2. A 20-year-old client with history of cryptorchidism
3. A 35-year-old male client complaining of scrotal pain and edema
4. A 55-year-old African American client with benign prostatic hypertrophy

ANSWER

3

RATIONALE

A male client complaining of scrotal pain and edema is more likely suffering from testicular torsion, requiring prompt assessment and intervention. If the condition is left untreated, infarction of the involved testes can occur.

REFERENCE

Nettina, S. M. (2007). *The Lippincott manual of nursing practice* (8th ed., Philippine ed.). Philadelphia: Lippincott Williams & Wilkins.

SUBJECT Renal Stone

CONCEPT
Clients with alkaline stones should be given an acid ash diet and clients with acid stones should be given an alkaline ash diet.

POINTERS
Acid ash diet
- Usually includes:

3P runes
lums
astries

3C heese
ranberry
orn

- Indicated for alkaline stones

Alkaline ash diet
- Usually includes milk
- Indicated for acid stones

QUESTION
Which of the following diets is appropriate for a client with calcium oxalate stones?

1. Acid ash
2. Alkaline ash
3. Gluten free
4. Purine free

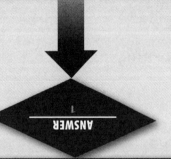

ANSWER
1

RATIONALE
An acid ash diet is an appropriate diet in a client with calcium oxalate and struvite stones due to their alkaline chemistry. Cystine stones require alkaline ash foods.

REFERENCE
Nettina, S. M. (2007). *The Lippincott manual of nursing practice* (8th ed., Philippine ed.). Philadelphia: Lippincott Williams & Wilkins.

NCLEX-RN CATEGORY **Basic Care and Comfort**

CONCEPT

Allopurinol inhibits uric acid production.

POINTERS

Allopurinol
- Used to prevent or treat attacks of gout
- Decreases uric acid levels
- Best taken with food
- Instruct the client to report sore throat.
- Increase fluid intake to facilitate excretion of uric acid crystals

Colchicine
- Decreases deposition of uric acid in the joints
- Common side effects include vomiting, diarrhea, abdominal pain, and peripheral neuritis

Probenecid
- Used as a uricosoric drug in gouty arthritis; delays the excretion of penicillin
- Decreases uric acid levels
- Best taken with meals
- Change position slowly
- Increase fluid intake

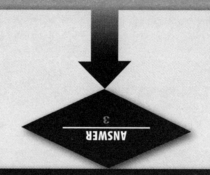

QUESTION

Which of the following is the primary purpose of allopurinol (Zyloprim) for a client with gout?

1. It promotes excretion of uric acid
2. It prevents inflammation
3. It decreases uric acid production
4. It prevents the deposition of uric acid in the joints

ANSWER

3

RATIONALE

Allopurinol decreases uric acid production in a client with gout.

REFERENCE

Karch, A. M. (2007). *2008 Lippincott's nursing drug guide.* Philadelphia: Lippincott Williams & Wilkins.

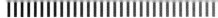

CONCEPT

Low-protein diet is indicated for clients with azotemia.

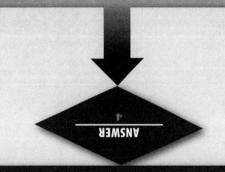

QUESTION

Which of the following foods is an appropriate selection for a client with azotemia?

1. Turkey sandwich with orange juice
2. Cheeseburger and sliced pears
3. Chicken sandwich with lettuce and tomato
4. Macaroni and vegetables

ANSWER

4

RATIONALE

The appropriate diet for a client with azotemia is a low-protein diet (e.g., macaroni and vegetables) to prevent accumulation of nitrogenous wastes in the body.

POINTERS

Azotemia
- Retention of metabolic waste products

Manifestations:
- Persistent nausea, vomiting
- Lethargy
- Uremic fetor (urine-smelling breath)
- Pruritus
- Hypertension

PRIORITY:
- Maintaining fluid balance

REFERENCE

Smeltzer, S. C., Bare, B. G., Hinkle, J. L., & Cheever, K. H. (2006). *Brunner and Suddarth's textbook of medical-surgical nursing.* Philadelphia: Lippincott Williams & Wilkins.

CONCEPT

Turner's syndrome is characterized by the absence of signs and symptoms of puberty.

QUESTION

Which of the following manifestation(s) is/are indicative of Turner's syndrome? Select all that apply.

1. Tall
2. Amenorrhea
3. Thin
4. Underdeveloped breasts
5. Mental retardation/intellectual disability
6. Absence of pubic hair

POINTERS

- Turner's syndrome was first described in 1938 by Dr. Henry Turner.
- Manifestations include short stature, webbing of the skin of the neck, low hairline at the back of the head, low set ears, drooping of the eyelids, breast underdevelopment, and a larger than usual number of moles on the skin.
- Diagnosed with a **karyotype test**.
- There is no cure for the condition.
- Treatment includes administration of growth hormones and estrogen replacement therapy.

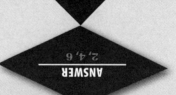

ANSWER

2, 4, 6

RATIONALE

Absence of signs and symptoms of puberty is indicative of Turner's syndrome, therefore a client with the disease will manifest amenorrhea, underdeveloped breasts, and an absence of pubic hair.

REFERENCE

Nettina, S. M. (2007). *The Lippincott manual of nursing practice* (8th ed., Philippine ed.). Philadelphia: Lippincott Williams & Wilkins.

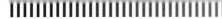

SUBJECT Desmopressin Acetate (Stimate)

CONCEPT

Desmopressin acetate is used in the treatment of von Willebrand's disease.

POINTERS

- Stimate may cause facial flushing.
- Monitor the nasal passages when using the nares in long-term therapy.
- Common side effects include:
  ▸ Gastric cramping
  ▸ Facial flushing
  ▸ Headache
  ▸ Nasal irritation
- Report drowsiness, shortness of breath, and headache.

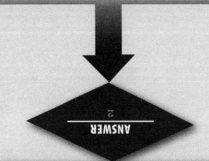

QUESTION

Desmopressin acetate (Stimate) is ordered for a client with von Willebrand's disease for which of the following reasons?

1. To promote reabsorption of water
2. To increase von Willebrand's factor
3. To treat chronic autonomic failure
4. To decrease nocturnal enuresis

ANSWER

2

RATIONALE

Stimate increases von Willebrand's factor, thereby increasing the levels of factor VIII and preventing bleeding.

REFERENCE
Karch, A. M. (2007). *2008 Lippincott's nursing drug guide*. Philadelphia: Lippincott Williams & Wilkins.

SUBJECT Metabolic Acidosis

CONCEPT

Metabolic acidosis is characterized by low pH and low bicarbonate levels.

POINTERS

- Causes of metabolic acidosis:
  - ▸ Ketone overproduction
  - ▸ Lactic acidosis
  - ▸ Kidney disorders
  - ▸ GI disorders like diarrhea
- Manifestations:
  Confusion
  Hypotension
  Anorexia
  Weakness
  Dull headache
  Kussmaul's breathing

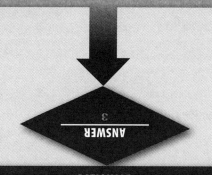

QUESTION

Which of the following laboratory data suggest metabolic acidosis?

1. Low pH and carbon dioxide levels
2. High pH and low carbon dioxide levels
3. Low pH and low bicarbonate levels
4. High pH and high bicarbonate levels

ANSWER

3

RATIONALE

Low pH and low bicarbonate levels are suggestive of metabolic acidosis.

REFERENCE

Nettina, S. M. (2007). *The Lippincott manual of nursing practice* (8th ed., Philippine ed.). Philadelphia: Lippincott Williams & Wilkins.

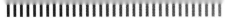

CONCEPT

Stress triggers Addisonian crisis.

POINTERS

- Addison's disease is caused by adrenal hypofunction, usually due to autoimmune disease.
- Common manifestations include hypotension and bronze skin pigmentation.
- It causes hyponatremia, hyperkalemia, and hypoglycemia.
- Monitor fluid and electrolyte balance.
- Explain the need for lifelong medications.
- Maintain a high sodium, low potassium diet.
- Advise the client to avoid infection, trauma, or stress, as these increase the risk for Addisonian crisis.

QUESTION

Which of the following instructions should a nurse provide a client with Addison's disease?

1. "Stop taking your steroids after you feel better."
2. "Make sure you take your steroids before visiting your dentist."
3. "Watching live concerts is a good way to decrease your stress."
4. "You may need to eat extra servings of fruits."

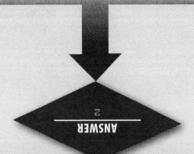

ANSWER

2

RATIONALE

Sources of stress include surgical procedures, infection, or development of other illness; hence the nurse should instruct the client to take steroids prior to visiting a dentist.

REFERENCE

Nettina, S. M. (2007). *The Lippincott manual of nursing practice* (8th ed., Philippine ed.). Philadelphia: Lippincott Williams & Wilkins.

CONCEPT

Obesity is the most prominent manifestation of Cushing's syndrome.

POINTERS

- Cushing's syndrome is caused by hypersecretion of glucocorticoids by the adrenal glands.
- It is common in females.
- Manifestations include:
  Central type obesity
  Unstable emotion (mood swings)
  Slender arms and legs
  Hirsutism in women
  Irritability
  No/decreased libido
  Gynecomastia in males
  Striae on the skin

QUESTION

Which of the following is/are the manifestation/s of Cushing's syndrome? Select all that apply.

1. Rounded face
2. Hypotension
3. Buffalo hump
4. Hypoglycemia
5. Weight gain
6. Bulking of skeletal muscles

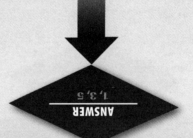

ANSWER

1, 3, 5

RATIONALE

A rounded face, buffalo hump, and obesity are among the clinical manifestations of Cushing's syndrome.

REFERENCE

Nettina, S. M. (2007). *The Lippincott manual of nursing practice* (8th ed., Philippine ed.). Philadelphia: Lippincott Williams & Wilkins.

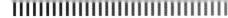

CONCEPT

Cushing's syndrome is characterized by:
- **Hypokalemia**
- **Hypernatremia**
- **Hyperglycemia**
- **Hypertension**

POINTERS
- In Cushing's syndrome, there is hypersecretion of glucocorticoids by the adrenal glands.
- Central type or truncal obesity with thin extremities, moon face, buffalo hump, and hirsutism occur.
- Maintain the client on a high potassium, low sodium diet.
- Instruct the client that treatment will involve lifelong administration of glucocorticoid synthesis inhibitors such as mitotane.
- Inform the client that there will be slow wound healing.

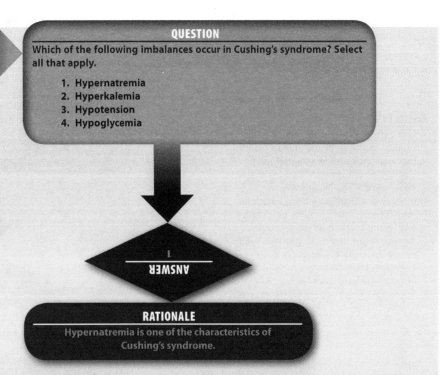

QUESTION

Which of the following imbalances occur in Cushing's syndrome? Select all that apply.

1. Hypernatremia
2. Hyperkalemia
3. Hypotension
4. Hypoglycemia

ANSWER

1

RATIONALE

Hypernatremia is one of the characteristics of Cushing's syndrome.

REFERENCE

Nettina, S. M. (2007). *The Lippincott manual of nursing practice* (8th ed., Philippine ed.). Philadelphia: Lippincott Williams & Wilkins.

CONCEPT

Most neuroendocrine conditions require lifetime medications.

POINTERS

- Cushing's syndrome is due to hypersecretion of glucocorticoids by the adrenal glands.
- Laboratory tests reveal elevated serum cortisol levels, hypernatremia, hypokalemia, hypertension, and hyperglycemia.
- Maintain the client on a high potassium (fruits), high protein (poultry products), low calorie, low carbohydrate (minimize bread, rice and cereal), low sodium (avoid preserved foods) diet to prevent edema and hypertension.
- Instruct the client that treatment will involve lifelong administration of glucocorticoid synthesis inhibitors such as mitotane.

QUESTION

Which of the following statements made by a client with Cushing's syndrome indicates to the nurse that further discharge teaching is needed for this client?

1. "I will look normal as treatment progresses."
2. "I will gradually discontinue my pills when I begin to feel better."
3. "I should check my blood pressure frequently."
4. "I can eat fruits."

ANSWER

2

RATIONALE

The client's statement "I will gradually discontinue the medication when I feel better" requires further instruction from the nurse because most neuroendocrine conditions require a lifetime intake of medication.

REFERENCE

Nettina, S. M. (2007). *The Lippincott manual of nursing practice* (8th ed., Philippine ed.). Philadelphia: Lippincott Williams & Wilkins.

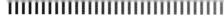

SUBJECT Hypoparathyroidism

CONCEPT

Hypoparathyroidism is characterized by decreased serum calcium and increased phosphorus levels.

POINTERS

- The most common cause of hypoparathyroidism is accidental removal of the parathyroid gland during thyroidectomy.
- Manifestations of hypoparathyroidism:
  - ▸ Tetany-general muscular hypertonia
  - ▸ Renal colic
  - ▸ Severe anxiety
- PRIORITY:
  - ▸ Administer calcium solution as prescribed
  - ▸ Note that too rapid administration of calcium leads to cardiac arrest

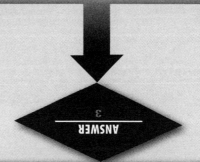

QUESTION

Which of the following conditions occurs in a client with hypoparathyroidism?

1. Decreased serum calcium and phosphorus levels
2. Increased serum calcium and phosphorus levels
3. Decreased serum calcium and increased phosphorus levels
4. Increased serum calcium and decreased phosphorus levels

ANSWER

3

RATIONALE

Hypoparathyroidism occurs in about 4% of clients due to accidental removal of parathyroid glands during thyroid surgery, resulting in hypocalcemia and hyperphosphatemia.

REFERENCE

Nettina, S. M. (2007). *The Lippincott manual of nursing practice* (8th ed., Philippine ed.). Philadelphia: Lippincott Williams & Wilkins.

214

CONCEPT

Trousseau's sign indicates hypocalcemia.

POINTERS

- A positive Trousseau's sign or carpopedal spasm is induced by occluding circulation in the arm with a blood pressure cuff.
- It is due to hypocalcemic tetany.

PRIORITY:

- Maintain a patent airway.
- Keep suction equipment and tracheostomy at the bedside.
- Administer IV calcium as directed.

QUESTION

A nurse was obtaining the blood pressure of a post-thyroidectomy client when she noticed that the client's fingers became spastic. This is due to a deficiency of:

1. Potassium
2. Calcium
3. Sodium
4. Magnesium

ANSWER

2

RATIONALE

Fingers becoming spastic during blood pressure taking is a positive indication of Trousseau's sign, which is indicative of hypocalcemia. Hypocalcemia is common in 4% of post-thyroidectomy clients whose parathyroid glands were accidentally removed during thyroid surgery.

REFERENCE

Nettina, S. M. (2007). *The Lippincott manual of nursing practice* (8th ed., Philippine ed.). Philadelphia: Lippincott Williams & Wilkins.

CONCEPT

When planning for client teaching programs, the nurse should first assess the client's knowledge.

POINTERS

- Diabetes mellitus is a chronic disorder of carbohydrate, protein, and fat metabolism characterized by an imbalance between insulin supply and demand.
- Polyuria, polydipsia, polyphagia, and weight loss are all signs of diabetes mellitus.
- Elevated FBS level is noted.
- Treatment includes:
  Diet: 50–60% cho, 20–30% fats, 10–20% chon
  Insulin
  Antidiabetic agents: Tolbutamide
  Blood sugar monitoring
  Exercise
  Transplant of the pancreas
  Ensure adequate food intake
  Scrupulous foot care
- Assess the client for Dawn phenomenon, an elevation of blood glucose between 5 am to 6 am due to nocturnal release of growth hormone. Treatment includes administration of intermediate acting insulin at 10 pm. Assess the client for rebound hyperglycemia or Somogyi phenomenon. Treatment includes adjusting the insulin dose.

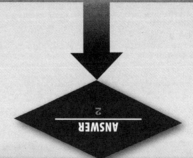

QUESTION

A nurse is planning a teaching program on foot care for a client with diabetes mellitus. What should the nurse do first?

1. Check on the client's educational background
2. Ask the client what she already knows about foot care
3. Provide the client with manuals on foot care
4. Refer the client for a group therapy session with clients having circulatory problems

ANSWER

2

RATIONALE

When planning a health teaching program, the nurse should initially assess the client's baseline knowledge regarding foot care.

REFERENCE

Nettina, S. M. (2007). *The Lippincott manual of nursing practice* (8th ed., Philippine ed.). Philadelphia: Lippincott Williams & Wilkins.

NCLEX-RN CATEGORY Physiological Adaptation

CONCEPT

Hypoglycemia induced by insulin usually occurs before meals.

QUESTION

After administration of regular insulin, when should the nurse expect the symptoms of hypoglycemia to occur?

1. Before dinner
2. Before breakfast the next day
3. At midnight
4. Before lunch

POINTERS

Signs and Symptoms of Hypoglycemia

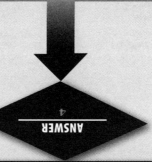

4D

iaphoresis
izziness
ecreased level of consciousness
ifficulty in problem solving

ANSWER

4

RATIONALE

Regular insulin peaks in 2 to 6 hours after administration. Hypoglycemia that occurs before lunch coincides with the peak of action of the regular insulin.

REFERENCE

Karch, A. M. (2007). *2008 Lippincott's nursing drug guide.* Philadelphia: Lippincott Williams & Wilkins.

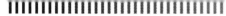

SUBJECT Rosiglitazone (Avandia)

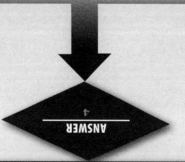

CONCEPT

Avandia is an antidiabetic agent.

QUESTION

Which of the following laboratory data should the nurse primarily monitor in a client who is receiving rosiglitazone (Avandia)?

1. Urine output
2. White blood cell count
3. Platelet count
4. Blood sugar levels

POINTERS

- In clients receiving Avandia, monitor glucose levels.
- May decrease effectiveness of contraceptives
- Report any of the following to the physician:
  ▸ Sore throat
  ▸ Bleeding
  ▸ Bruising
  ▸ Light-colored stools

ANSWER

4

RATIONALE

Avandia is an antidiabetic agent that stimulates insulin receptor sites to lower blood glucose and improve the action of insulin. Therefore, blood sugar levels should be monitored carefully.

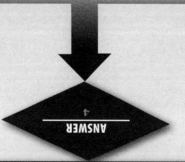

REFERENCE

Karch, A. M. (2007). *2008 Lippincott's nursing drug guide.* Philadelphia: Lippincott Williams & Wilkins.

CONCEPT

Removal of the pituitary gland leads to infertility.

POINTERS

Nursing care principles for clients post hypophysectomy

Head of the bed should be elevated
Evaluate vital signs, the level of consciousness, and neurological status
Avoid sneezing, coughing, and blowing the nose
Diabetes insipidus, manifested by polyuria, may occur due to antidiuretic hormone disturbances

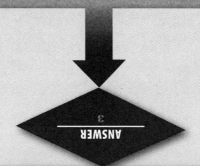

QUESTION

Hypophysectomy will possibly cause emotional difficulty in which of the following clients?

1. A 45-year-old postmenopausal female
2. A 30-year-old multipara female
3. A 25-year-old newlywed female
4. A 50-year-old male

ANSWER

3

RATIONALE

A 25-year-old newlywed female client may encounter emotional difficulties, because hypophysectomy could lead to infertility.

REFERENCE

Nettina, S. M. (2007). *The Lippincott manual of nursing practice* (8th ed., Philippine ed.). Philadelphia: Lippincott Williams & Wilkins.

SUBJECT Thyroid Crisis

CONCEPT

Elevated temperature and heart rate after thyroid surgery indicate thyroid crisis.

POINTERS

Manifestations of thyroid crisis

High fever (above 38.5 °C)
Exaggerated manifestations of
hyperthyroidism
Altered neurologic function
Tachycardia (more than 130 beats/minute)

- Thyroid crisis is usually precipitated by:
  ▸ Stress
  ▸ Injury
  ▸ Infection
  ▸ Tooth extraction

- PRIORITY: Provide a cool environment

QUESTION

Which of the following should be the priority goals of care for clients after thyroid surgery? Select all that apply.

1. To decrease body temperature
2. To promote bowel elimination
3. To increase urine output
4. To prevent joint contracture deformity
5. To decrease the heart rate

ANSWER

1, 5

RATIONALE

An elevated temperature and heart rate after thyroid surgery are indicative of thyroid crisis.

REFERENCE

Nettina, S. M. (2007). *The Lippincott manual of nursing practice* (8th ed., Philippine ed.). Philadelphia: Lippincott Williams & Wilkins.

220

CONCEPT

Urine is the major source of contamination for clients treated with radioactive iodine 131.

POINTERS

- Iodine 131 is an antithyroid; it limits thyroid hormone secretion.
- Normal heart rate and adequate sleep indicate effective treatment.
- Instruct client to fast overnight before administration as food delays absorption.
- It will take several weeks (usually 6) before therapeutic effects become noticeable.
- Urine and saliva are slightly radioactive for 24 hours after administration.

QUESTION

After the administration of radioactive iodine 131 to a client, the nurse should be careful in handling which of the following? Select all that apply.

1. Blood
2. Sputum
3. Bedpans
4. Urinals
5. Linens

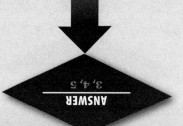

ANSWER

3, 4, 5

RATIONALE

Radioactive iodine is highly toxic, therefore any materials that might have been contaminated by a client's urine should be handled carefully.

REFERENCE

Gapuz, R. *The ABCs of passing foreign nursing exams*. Philippines: Gapuz Publications.

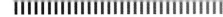

CONCEPT

PTU inhibits synthesis of thyroid hormone.

POINTERS

- PTU is an antithyroid; it inhibits synthesis of thyroid hormone.
- It decreases heart rate and promotes adequate sleep.
- Take the drug around the clock at 8 hour intervals.
- Treatment is lifelong.
- Report the development of a sore throat to the physician; it indicates agranulocytosis.
- Monitor the heart rate; PTU causes tachycardia.
- PTU is contraindicated in pregnant clients.

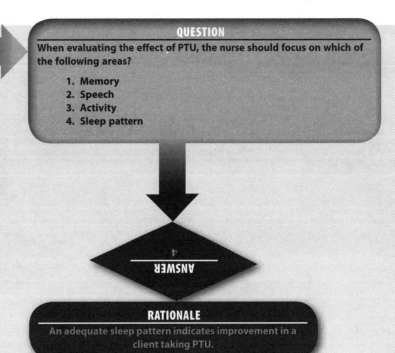

QUESTION

When evaluating the effect of PTU, the nurse should focus on which of the following areas?

1. Memory
2. Speech
3. Activity
4. Sleep pattern

ANSWER

4

RATIONALE

An adequate sleep pattern indicates improvement in a client taking PTU.

REFERENCE

Karch, A. M. (2007). *2008 Lippincott's nursing drug guide*. Philadelphia: Lippincott Williams & Wilkins.

CONCEPT

Tapazole blocks autonomic nervous system reactions.

222

POINTERS

- Take Tapazole around the clock at 8 hour intervals.

Common side effects include:
- Dizziness
- Weakness
- Drowsiness
- Vertigo
- Vomiting
- Anorexia
- Rash
- Itching

Report to the physician:
- Fever
- Sore throat
- Unusual bleeding
- Bruising
- Headache
- Body malaise

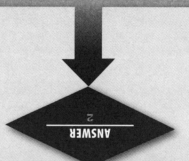

QUESTION

Which of the following questions should the nurse ask to evaluate the effectiveness of Tapazole therapy in a client with hyperthyroidism?

1. "Have you noticed any improvement in your vision?"
2. "Has your pulse rate decreased?"
3. "Do you eat better now?"
4. "Do you still have difficulty sleeping?"

ANSWER

2

RATIONALE

A decrease in the pulse rate indicates blocking of the autonomic nervous system, the expected effect of Tapazole.

REFERENCE

Karch, A. M. (2007). *2008 Lippincott's nursing drug guide*. Philadelphia: Lippincott Williams & Wilkins.

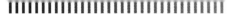

SUBJECT Hypomagnesemia

CONCEPT
Polyuria decreases magnesium levels.

POINTERS
- Magnesium facilitates smooth muscle regulation.
- The normal RDA is 280–350 mg.
- Manifestations of hypomagnesemia:
  - ▸ Tetany
  - ▸ Tremors
  - ▸ Tachycardia
  - ▸ Depression
  - ▸ Seizures
  - ▸ Dysrhythmias
- Sources of magnesium include nuts, meat, green vegetables, seafood, and dairy products.

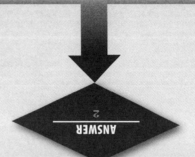

QUESTION
Which of the following questions may lead the nurse to identify a predisposing factor for hypomagnesemia?

1. "Are you taking calcium supplements?"
2. "Do you have diabetes mellitus?"
3. "Do you have any bowel problems?"
4. "Did you have a thyroid surgery recently?"

ANSWER
2

RATIONALE
A client with diabetes mellitus exhibits polyuria, which puts the client at risk of developing hypomagnesemia.

REFERENCE
Nettina, S. M. (2007). *The Lippincott manual of nursing practice* (8th ed., Philippine ed.). Philadelphia: Lippincott Williams & Wilkins.

CONCEPT

When phosphorus level goes up, calcium level goes down and vice versa.

POINTERS

- Phosphorus facilitates nerve and muscle activity, bone and tooth formation, and RBC production.
- The RDA is 800 to 1,200 mg.
- Causes of hyperphosphatemia:
  ▸ Renal failure (most common)
  ▸ Hypoparathyroidism
  ▸ Chemotherapy
  ▸ Muscle necrosis
  ▸ Increased phosphorus absorption
- Clinical manifestations:
  ▸ Tetany
  ▸ Seizure
  ▸ Renal damage
- Sources of phosphate include eggs, fish, yellow cheese, almonds, chocolate, peanut, rye, and wheat.

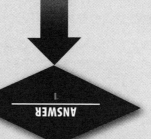

QUESTION

Which of the following data in a client's history is related to hyperphosphatemia?

1. Thyroid surgery
2. Gastric surgery
3. Rectal surgery
4. Renal surgery

ANSWER

1

RATIONALE

Hypoparathyroidism occurs in about 4% of clients due to accidental removal of the parathyroid glands during thyroid surgery. Hypoparathyroidism leads to hypocalcemia and hyperphosphatemia.

REFERENCE

Nettina, S. M. (2007). *The Lippincott manual of nursing practice* (8th ed., Philippine ed.). Philadelphia: Lippincott Williams & Wilkins.

CONCEPT

Acromegaly is characterized by irreversible increase of the digits of the hands and feet.

POINTERS

- Acromegaly is due to over-secretion of growth hormone.
- It is characterized by coarsening of facial features and increased shoe size.
- Serum human growth hormone and blood sugar levels are elevated.
- Provide emotional support.
- Prepare the client for surgery.
- Monitor for signs and symptoms of diabetes.

QUESTION

Which of these questions is appropriate for the nurse to ask a client who is suspected of having acromegaly?

1. "Do you urinate often at night?"
2. "Are you buying larger size shoes?"
3. "Is your mouth frequently dry after meals?"
4. "Did you have alopecia lately?"

ANSWER

2

RATIONALE

Frequent shoe size changes, due to enlarging digits, is indicative of having acromegaly.

REFERENCE

Gapuz, R. *The ABCs of passing foreign nursing exams.* Philippines: Gapuz Publications.

SUBJECT Syndrome of Inappropriate Antidiuretic Hormone Secretion (SIADH)

CONCEPT

SIADH causes fluid retention.

POINTERS

- SIADH may occur in clients with lung cancer, severe pneumonia, pneumothorax, lead poisoning, brain surgery, tumors, or infection.
- SIADH leads to dilutional hyponatremia.
- PRIORITY:
  - ▶ Fluid restriction
  - ▶ Daily weight monitoring
  - ▶ Monitoring of urine, blood chemistries, and neurologic status

QUESTION

Which of these manifestations suggests the development of a complication in a client with syndrome of inappropriate antidiuretic hormone secretion (SIADH)?

1. Polyuria
2. Weight loss
3. Distended neck veins
4. Muscle rigidity

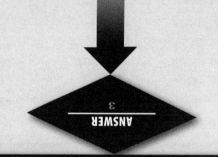

ANSWER

3

RATIONALE

SIADH causes vascular overload, usually manifested by neck vein distention.

REFERENCE

Nettina, S. M. (2007). *The Lippincott manual of nursing practice* (8th ed., Philippine ed.). Philadelphia: Lippincott Williams & Wilkins.

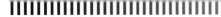

SUBJECT Vasopressin (Pitressin)

CONCEPT

Pitressin increases the specific gravity of the urine.

POINTERS

Pitressin promotes reabsorption of water.
Common side effects include:

- Tremors
- Sweating
- Vertigo
- Vomiting

Report any of the following to the physician:

- Drowsiness
- Light-headedness
- Headache
- Coma
- Convulsions

These indicate **water intoxication**.

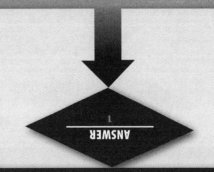

QUESTION

A client with diabetes insipidus is receiving vasopressin (Pitressin). Which of the following findings indicates that the drug is exerting its therapeutic effect?

1. The urine becomes more concentrated
2. The urine becomes light yellow
3. The urine becomes alkaline
4. The urine output increases in amount

ANSWER

1

RATIONALE

An increase in the specific gravity of the urine indicates the ability of the kidney to concentrate the urine, which is a positive outcome of the use of Pitressin.

REFERENCE
Karch, A. M. (2007). *2008 Lippincott's nursing drug guide*. Philadelphia: Lippincott Williams & Wilkins.

227

NCLEX-RN CATEGORY **Pharmacological and Parenteral Therapies**

SUBJECT Cushing's Triad

CONCEPT

Cushing's triad indicates increased intracranial pressure (ICP).

POINTERS

Nursing care of clients with increased ICP

Head of the bed should be elevated
Evaluate level of consciousness
Airway maintenance
Decrease cerebral edema by administering
diuretics and corticosteroids

QUESTION

An elevated blood pressure, decreased heart rate, and decreased respiratory rate are commonly found in clients with which of the following conditions?

1. Shock
2. Increased intracranial pressure
3. Pericarditis
4. Heart failure

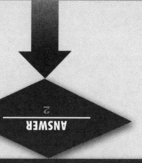

ANSWER

2

RATIONALE

Cushing's triad, consisting of elevated blood pressure, decreased respiratory rate, and decreased heart rate, indicates increased intracranial pressure.

REFERENCE

Nettina, S. M. (2007). *The Lippincott manual of nursing practice* (8th ed., Philippine ed.). Philadelphia: Lippincott Williams & Wilkins.

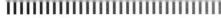

SUBJECT Magnetic Resonance Imaging (MRI)

CONCEPT

Metal objects are not allowed in clients for MRI.

POINTERS

- MRI provides cross-sectional images of brain tissues that are more detailed than a CT scan.
- Contraindications include pregnant women, obesity (more than 300 lbs.), claustrophobic clients, clients with unstable vital signs, and clients with metal implants like a pacemaker, hip replacement, or jewelry.

QUESTION

Which of the following questions should the nurse ask a client who is scheduled for magnetic resonance imaging?

1. "Did you have hip replacement surgery?"
2. "Do you have a history of sore throat?"
3. "Can you tolerate a fatty meal?"
4. "Do you have any history of trauma?"

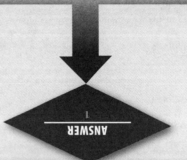

ANSWER

1

RATIONALE

Prior to the MRI procedure, the nurse should remove all metal from the client and report the presence of any metal implants to the physician.

REFERENCE

Nettina, S. M. (2007). *The Lippincott manual of nursing practice* (8th ed., Philippine ed.). Philadelphia: Lippincott Williams & Wilkins.

NCLEX-RN CATEGORY **Reduction of Risk Potential**

CONCEPT

In bladder training, the most significant factor is regularity.

POINTERS

- Spinal cord injury involves partial or complete disruption of nerve tracts and neurons, resulting in paralysis and sensory loss.
- Paralysis depends on the level of injury:
  - ▸ Cervical: Quadriplegia
  - ▸ Thoracic: Paraplegia
  - ▸ Lumbar: Paraplegia
- X-ray reveals the location and extent of injury.
- Avoid hyperflexion and hyperextension of the spine. Log-roll the client.
- Keep a catheter at the bedside to prevent bladder distention, which may stimulate autonomic dysreflexia.

QUESTION

A client is undergoing rehabilitation after spinal cord injury. Which of the following discharge instructions should the nurse tell the client?

1. "Minimize your fluid intake to prevent nocturia."
2. "Make sure that you empty your bladder as scheduled."
3. "Increase your intake of cranberry juice."
4. "Avoid soda at all times."

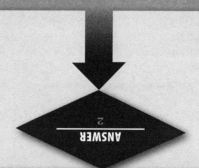

ANSWER

2

RATIONALE

Clients with spinal cord injury should establish a regular schedule of voiding (every 2–3 hours) because the most significant factor in bladder training is regularity.

REFERENCE

Nettina, S. M. (2007). *The Lippincott manual of nursing practice* (8th ed., Philippine ed.). Philadelphia: Lippincott Williams & Wilkins.

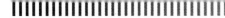

CONCEPT

The cerebellum maintains balance, gait, and coordination.

POINTERS

Assessing cerebellar function

- Cerebellar function is assessed to screen for coordination.
- Observe for posture and gait by asking the client to walk back and forth in a straight line.
- Instruct the client to run his heel down his left shin and vice versa for muscle coordination in the lower extremities.

QUESTION

Which of the following measures is a priority for a client with a cerebellar tumor?

1. Providing assistance with ambulation
2. Facilitating retention of facts by repeating instructions
3. Placing the client in a darkened room
4. Speaking slowly and clearly

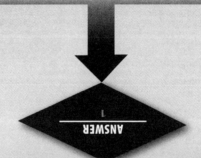

ANSWER

1

RATIONALE

The cerebellum maintains balance, gait, and coordination, therefore these are impaired in a client with a cerebellar tumor. The client will require assistance with ambulation to prevent injuries and accidents.

REFERENCE

Nettina, S. M. (2007). *The Lippincott manual of nursing practice* (8th ed., Philippine ed.). Philadelphia: Lippincott Williams & Wilkins.

231

NCLEX-RN CATEGORY **Management of Care**

CONCEPT

Canes should be handled on the stronger side of the body.

QUESTION

Which of the following discharge instructions on the use of a cane is/are appropriate for the nurse to give a client? Select all that apply.

1. Hold the cane 6 inches lateral to the base of the fifth toe
2. Handle the cane on the affected side
3. Flex the elbow at 30°
4. When going up the stairs, step up on the unaffected extremity, then place the cane and the affected extremity on the step
5. Make sure that the handle of the cane is approximately at the level of the greater trochanter

POINTERS

Use of a cane

- Hold the cane 6 inches lateral to the base of the fifth toe.
- The handle is approximately at the level of the greater trochanter.
- Handle the cane on the unaffected side.
- When going up the stairs, step up on the unaffected leg, then place the cane and affected extremity on the step.

ANSWER

1, 3, 4, 5

RATIONALE

Hold the cane in the hand opposite to the affected extremity (i.e. the cane should be used on the good side) to allow partial weight-bearing relief because the cane is in contact with the floor at the same time as the affected extremity.

REFERENCE

Nettina, S. M. (2007). *The Lippincott manual of nursing practice* (8th ed., Philippine ed.). Philadelphia: Lippincott Williams & Wilkins.

NCLEX-RN CATEGORY **Basic Care and Comfort**

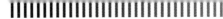

CONCEPT

The frontal lobe controls the motor speech area and personality.

QUESTION

Which of the following functions are attributed to the frontal lobe? Select all that apply.

1. Motor control
2. Ability to speak words
3. Sensation
4. Concentration
5. Memory
6. Judgment

POINTERS

Lobes of the brain

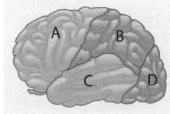

A. Frontal lobe
- Broca's motor speech area, language
- Motor functions/movements
- Control of morals, emotions, judgment, personality, concentration, problem solving, impulse control, reasoning, and planning

B. Parietal lobe
- Pain interpretation
- Sensation (touch, temperature, pressure, taste)
- Reading and arithmetic

C. Temporal lobe
- Auditory center/hearing
- Memory, perception, and recognition
- Wernickes' language area

D. Occipital lobe
- Visual processing

ANSWER

1, 2, 4, 5, 6

RATIONALE

Motor control, ability to speak words, concentration, memory, and judgment are all functions attributed to the frontal lobe of the brain.

REFERENCE

Nettina, S. M. (2007). *The Lippincott manual of nursing practice* (8th ed., Philippine ed.). Philadelphia: Lippincott Williams & Wilkins.

233

NCLEX-RN CATEGORY Reduction of Risk Potential

SUBJECT Lindane (Kwell)

CONCEPT

Kwell is neurotoxic.

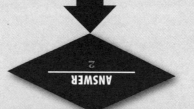

QUESTION

Kwell is contraindicated in which of the following clients?

1. A 50-year-old with a gastric ulcer
2. A 20-year-old with seizures
3. A 30-year-old newlywed
4. A 15-year-old with acne

POINTERS

- Kwell is considered effective if there are no lice on the hair and there are no eggs attached to hair shafts.
- Kwell is applied twice: immediately after diagnosis and a week later.
- May be administered to all individuals living in the house.
- Do not apply to the face.
- Use gloves to remove nits by using a fine-toothed comb rinsed in vinegar.

ANSWER

2

RATIONALE

Kwell is neurotoxic, therefore it is contraindicated in clients with seizure disorders.

REFERENCE

Karch, A. M. (2007). *2008 Lippincott's nursing drug guide.* Philadelphia: Lippincott Williams & Wilkins.

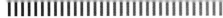
CONCEPT

Providing a quiet environment is the most important intervention for a client with bacterial meningitis.

POINTERS

Nursing care for clients with bacterial meningitis

- Isolate the client for 24 hours after the start of antibiotic therapy.
- Rifampicin is most commonly used for chemoprophylaxis for healthcare workers, household contacts in the community, and day care centers.
- Deafness may result as a complication in children; the parents should therefore be referred to an audiologist.
- For prevention of meningitis, ensure administration of HiB vaccine.

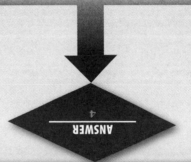

QUESTION

Which type of room is appropriate for a client with bacterial meningitis?

1. A well-lit room
2. A bright and cheerful room
3. A room near the nurse's station
4. A room that is quiet and dark

ANSWER

4

RATIONALE

Maintain a quiet, calm, and darkened environment for a client with bacterial meningitis to prevent seizures, which may cause an increase in intracranial pressure.

REFERENCE

Nettina, S. M. (2007). *The Lippincott manual of nursing practice* (8th ed., Philippine ed.). Philadelphia: Lippincott Williams & Wilkins.

CONCEPT

Pick's disease is a cognitive problem.

236

POINTERS

- Pick's disease is a degenerative brain illness.
- It usually begins after the age of 40.
- Manifestations:
  - ▸ **P**ersonality changes
  - ▸ **I**nappropriate sexual advances
  - ▸ **C**onfusion
  - ▸ **K**nowledge gaps/poor judgment
  - ▸ **S**peech/language difficulties

QUESTION

Which of the following indicates a sign of the beginning of Pick's disease?

1. Personality changes
2. Incontinence
3. Wandering with amnesia
4. Apraxia

ANSWER

1

RATIONALE

Pick's disease is a degenerative disorder initially manifested by personality changes. Incontinence, apraxia and wandering with amnesia occur later in the disorder.

REFERENCE

Nettina, S. M. (2007). *The Lippincott manual of nursing practice* (8th ed., Philippine ed.). Philadelphia: Lippincott Williams & Wilkins.

NCLEX-RN CATEGORY Psychosocial Integrity

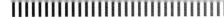

SUBJECT Parkinson's Disease

CONCEPT

Parkinson's disease is a degenerative disease characterized by abnormal motor function and failure of body systems.

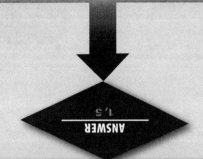

QUESTION

Which of the following manifestations are found in Parkinson's disease? Select all that apply.

1. Mask-like face
2. Intentional tremors
3. Rapid movement
4. Dry mouth
5. Dysphagia

POINTERS

Manifestations of Parkinson's disease:

Bradykinesia (slow movement)
Aching shoulders and arm
Drooling/excessive salivation

Difficulty swallowing and speaking
Extensive loss of coordination
Blank facial expression
Tremors (resting)

ANSWER

1, 5

RATIONALE

Mask-like faces and dysphagia are among the manifestations of Parkinson's disease. Intentional tremors are associated with multiple sclerosis.

REFERENCE

Nettina, S. M. (2007). *The Lippincott manual of nursing practice* (8th ed., Philippine ed.). Philadelphia: Lippincott Williams & Wilkins.

NCLEX-RN CATEGORY Physiological Adaptation

CONCEPT

Unilateral neglect occurs when a person cannot attend to or ignores the hemiplegic side of his body.

POINTERS

- Place the call light, television, telephone, and personal items on the unaffected side.
- The client's bed should be positioned so the unaffected side is toward the door.
- Approach the client from the unaffected side.
- Place food on the unaffected side of the mouth.

QUESTION

In a client with unilateral neglect due to right cerebral stroke, which nursing diagnosis is appropriate?

1. Risk for injury related to inability to perceive the upper part of the body
2. Risk for injury related to inability to perceive the right side of the body
3. Risk for injury related to inability to perceive the left side of the body
4. Risk for injury related to inability to perceive the lower part of the body

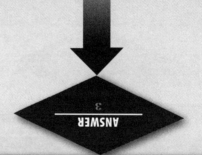

ANSWER

3

RATIONALE

A client with right cerebral stroke will manifest left-sided paralysis, therefore risk for injury related to inability to perceive the left side of the body is the appropriate nursing diagnosis.

REFERENCE

Carpenito-Moyet, L. J. (2007). *Handbook of nursing diagnosis* (12th ed.). Philadelphia: Lippincott Williams & Wilkins.

CONCEPT

Marfan's syndrome is characterized by spiderlike extremities.

QUESTION

An appropriate nursing diagnosis for a client with Marfan's syndrome is?

1. The client is at risk for injury
2. The client is in pain
3. The client has altered elimination
4. The client has altered nutrition

POINTERS

- Marfan's syndrome is an inherited abnormal condition (autosomal dominant trait) characterized by elongation of the bones, often with associated abnormalities of the eyes and the cardiovascular system. It affects men and women equally.
- There is muscular underdevelopment, joint hypermobility, and bone elongation (spiderlike extremities).
- There is no specific treatment.
- PRIORITY: Safety, prevent complications
- Common complications include aneurysm, dislocation of the lens of the eyes, and kyphoscoliosis.

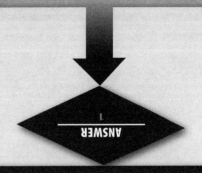

ANSWER

1

RATIONALE

Clients with Marfan's syndrome are at risk for injury due to muscular underdevelopment and joint hypermobility.

REFERENCE

Nettina, S. M. (2007). *The Lippincott manual of nursing practice* (8th ed., Philippine ed.). Philadelphia: Lippincott Williams & Wilkins.

239

NCLEX-RN CATEGORY Physiological Adaptation

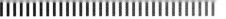

SUBJECT AIDS Dementia Complex/HIV

NCLEX-RN CATEGORY Physiological Adaptation

CONCEPT

AIDS dementia complex is characterized by unsteady gait and lack of coordination.

POINTERS

AIDS dementia complex

- Early manifestations:
  Forgetfulness
  Reduced concentration
  Ataxia, apathy, agitation
  Clumsiness
  Slowed movement
- Late manifestations:
  ▸ Paraplegia
  ▸ Vegetative state
  ▸ Mutism
- Treated with antiretroviral therapy that penetrate the central nervous system, such as Zidovudine (AZT), Stavudine hydroxyurea (d4T), Nevirapine (Viramune), and Abacovir.

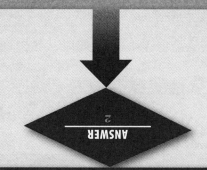

QUESTION

Which of the following interventions is appropriate for a client with AIDS dementia complex?

1. Provide various activities
2. Assist the client with ambulation
3. Increase exercise activities
4. Minimize reminders

ANSWER

2

RATIONALE

Assisting the client with ambulation is an appropriate nursing intervention because clients with AIDS dementia complex have an unsteady gait and suffer from a lack of coordination.

REFERENCE

Smeltzer, S. C., Bare, B. G., Hinkle, J. L., & Cheever, K. H. (2006). *Brunner and Suddarth's textbook of medical-surgical nursing.* Philadelphia: Lippincott Williams & Wilkins.

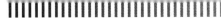

SUBJECT Carbamazepine (Tegretol)

CONCEPT

Tegretol causes pancytopenia.

POINTERS

- Tegretol is an antiepileptic agent.
- It is hepatotoxic and can cause fatal hepatitis.
- Administer the drug with food.
- Report bruising, unusual bleeding, sore throat, rash, and jaundice to the physician.

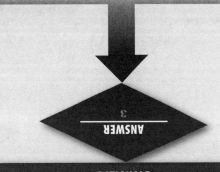

QUESTION

Which of the following laboratory data needs to be checked in a client who is taking carbamazepine (Tegretol)?

1. Serum electrolytes
2. Urinalysis
3. Complete blood count
4. Serum protein levels

ANSWER

3

RATIONALE

The client's CBC should be checked periodically because the drug can cause pancytopenia.

241

REFERENCE

Karch, A. M. (2007). *2008 Lippincott's nursing drug guide.* Philadelphia: Lippincott Williams & Wilkins.

NCLEX-RN CATEGORY **Pharmacological and Parenteral Therapies**

242

CONCEPT

Gingival hyperplasia is a common side effect of Dilantin.

POINTERS

- Therapeutic serum level of Dilantin is 10–20 ug/dL.
- Administer with food to enhance absorption.
- Discontinue if any of the following occur:
  - ▸ Measles-like rash
  - ▸ Enlarged lymph node
  - ▸ Hypersensitivity reaction
  - ▸ Hepatotoxicity
  - ▸ Bone marrow depression

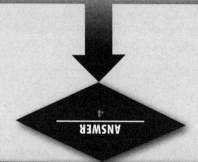

QUESTION

Which of the following interventions is appropriate for a client receiving phenytoin (Dilantin)?

1. Administer on an empty stomach
2. Tell the client that a measles-like rash is a normal side effect
3. Reassure the client that serum level monitoring is not necessary
4. Massage the gums

ANSWER

4

RATIONALE

A common side effect of phenytoin is gingival hyperplasia, hence the need to massage the gums, maintain good oral hygiene, and obtain frequent dental checkups to prevent serious gum disease.

REFERENCE

Karch, A. M. (2007). *2008 Lippincott's nursing drug guide.* Philadelphia: Lippincott Williams & Wilkins.

CONCEPT

Guillain-Barré syndrome leads to respiratory depression.

POINTERS

- Guillain-Barré syndrome is an acquired acute inflammatory disease of peripheral nerves.
- It causes ascending paralysis.
- CSF exam reveals elevated total protein.
- Maintain a patent airway.
- Instruct the client to avoid crowded areas.
- Keep tracheostomy at the bedside.

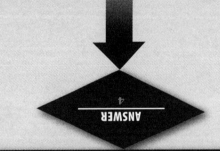

QUESTION

When assessing a client with Guillain-Barré syndrome, the nurse should focus on which of the following body systems?

1. Renal
2. Cardiovascular
3. Musculoskeletal
4. Respiratory

ANSWER

4

RATIONALE

A life-threatening complication of Guillain-Barré syndrome is respiratory failure due to weakness or paralysis of respiratory muscles.

243

NCLEX-RN CATEGORY **Reduction of Risk Potential**

REFERENCE

Nettina, S. M. (2007). *The Lippincott manual of nursing practice* (8th ed., Philippine ed.). Philadelphia: Lippincott Williams & Wilkins.

SUBJECT Amyotrophic Lateral Sclerosis (ALS)/Lou Gehrig's Disease

CONCEPT
Dysphagia is a common manifestation of ALS.

QUESTION
Which of the following nursing diagnoses is a priority for a client with amyotrophic lateral sclerosis (ALS)?

1. Impaired physical mobility
2. Altered tissue perfusion
3. Risk for aspiration
4. Social isolation

POINTERS
Manifestations of ALS

Atrophy of muscles, fasciculations, and spasticity
Lower extremities become weak
Swallowing and speaking difficulties

Common complications:

Aspiration pneumonia
Respiratory failure
Cardiovascular arrest

ANSWER
3

RATIONALE
In ALS, there is progressive difficulty in swallowing (drooling, regurgitation of liquids through the nose) and ultimately in breathing, putting the client at risk for aspiration.

REFERENCE
Nettina, S. M. (2007). *The Lippincott manual of nursing practice* (8th ed., Philippine ed.). Philadelphia: Lippincott Williams & Wilkins.

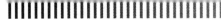

SUBJECT Myasthenia Gravis

CONCEPT

Difficulty in swallowing is a common sign of myasthenia gravis.

QUESTION

Which activity is contraindicated for a client with myasthenia gravis before meals?

1. Deep breathing and coughing exercises
2. Range of motion exercises
3. Talking for long periods over the phone
4. Watching TV

POINTERS

- Myasthenia gravis is characterized by faulty neuromuscular transmission of the voluntary muscles of the body due to a deficiency in acetylcholine receptor sites in the myoneural junction.
- Characterized by descending muscle weakness initially manifested by ptosis.
- CT scan reveals hyperplasia of the thymus gland.
- Tensilon test: increased muscle strength 30 seconds after administration of edrophonium.
- Maintain patent airway.
- Instruct the client to avoid quinidine, morphine, and antibiotics since these may trigger muscle weakness.
- Instruct the client to avoid prolonged talking over the phone especially before meals since this will weaken the facial muscles that are used for eating.

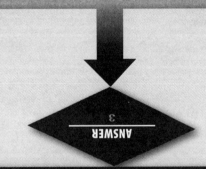

ANSWER

3

RATIONALE

Clients with myasthenia gravis should be instructed to speak in a slow manner to avoid voice strain. The nurse should stress the importance of scheduled rest periods before meals since the muscles used for eating can be weakened by continuous talking activity.

REFERENCE

Nettina, S. M. (2007). *The Lippincott manual of nursing practice* (8th ed., Philippine ed.). Philadelphia: Lippincott Williams & Wilkins.

SUBJECT Diazepam (Valium)

CONCEPT

Valium can cause respiratory depression.

POINTERS

- Valium is an antianxiety drug and is given as a muscle relaxant to clients in traction.
- It is best taken before meals as food in the stomach delays absorption.
- Avoid the intake of alcohol and caffeine-containing foods, since these alter the effects of the drug.
- Administer it separately because it is incompatible with any drug.
- It should not be given when a client is taking valerian, kava kava, or herbal sedatives.

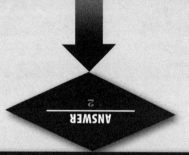

QUESTION

Which of the following drugs is contraindicated in clients with myasthenia gravis?

1. Neostigmine
2. Valium
3. Lasix
4. Mannitol

ANSWER

2

RATIONALE

A complication of myasthenia gravis is respiratory failure due to paralysis of the respiratory muscles. Administration of valium is contraindicated because it causes respiratory depression.

REFERENCE

Karch, A. M. (2007). *2008 Lippincott's nursing drug guide*. Philadelphia: Lippincott Williams & Wilkins.

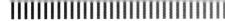

SUBJECT Guillain-Barré Syndrome

CONCEPT

Ascending paralysis occurs in Guillain-Barré syndrome.

POINTERS

- Guillain-Barré syndrome is an acquired acute inflammatory disease of peripheral nerves.
- It causes ascending paralysis.
- CSF exam reveals elevated total protein.
- Maintain a patent airway.
- Instruct the client to avoid crowded areas.
- Keep tracheostomy at the bedside.

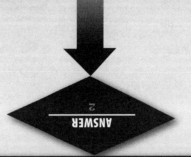

QUESTION

Which of the following manifestations of Guillain-Barré syndrome indicates a need for further assessment?

1. Decreasing leg strength
2. Decreasing voice volume
3. Muscle weakness in the legs
4. Dragging sensation in the arms

ANSWER

2

RATIONALE

A decrease in voice volume indicates progressive ascending neuropathy towards the laryngeal area. This can possibly lead to breathing difficulty.

REFERENCE

Nettina, S. M. (2007). *The Lippincott manual of nursing practice* (8th ed., Philippine ed.). Philadelphia: Lippincott Williams & Wilkins.

NCLEX-RN CATEGORY Reduction of Risk Potential

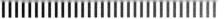
CONCEPT

Neurogenic shock is characterized by areflexia (absence of reflexes).

248

POINTERS

- Spinal shock ends when reflexes are regained.
- Assess the reflex, motor, sensory, and autonomic activity below the level of the lesion.
- Maintain pulmonary and cardiovascular stability.

QUESTION

Which of the following manifestations are found in clients with neurogenic shock? Select all that apply.

1. Muscle paralysis
2. Flaccid paralysis
3. Hypotension
4. Bradycardia
5. Paralytic ileus

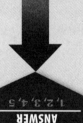

ANSWER

1, 2, 3, 4, 5

RATIONALE

Neurogenic shock develops due to the loss of autonomic nervous system function below the level of the lesion, causing blood pressure and heart rate to fall, which leads to low cardiac output and peripheral vasodilation.

REFERENCE

Smeltzer, S. C., Bare, B. G., Hinkle, J. L., & Cheever, K. H. (2006). *Brunner and Suddarth's textbook of medical-surgical nursing.* Philadelphia: Lippincott Williams & Wilkins.

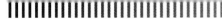

CONCEPT

Autonomic dysreflexia is triggered by a full bladder or bowels.

POINTERS

- Autonomic dysreflexia occurs after a spinal cord injury at the level of T6 or above.
- It may result in dangerously elevated blood pressure.
- Common causes:
  Bladder and bowel distention
  Obstructions (kidney stone) and constrictions (clothing, shoes, apparatus)
  Bowel impaction
  Strong odors, pain, pressure
- Common manifestations include a pounding headache, profuse sweating, and piloerection (3 Ps)
- PRIORITY: Sit the client up and assess for bladder patency.

QUESTION

Which of the following equipment should the nurse prepare at the bedside of a client with autonomic dysreflexia?

1. Tracheostomy set
2. Endotracheal tube
3. Tourniquet
4. Catheterization set

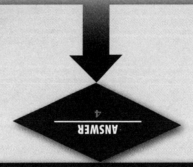

ANSWER

4

RATIONALE

The nurse should prepare a catheterization set at the bedside because autonomic dysreflexia is triggered by bladder distention.

REFERENCE

Nettina, S. M. (2007). *The Lippincott manual of nursing practice* (8th ed., Philippine ed.). Philadelphia: Lippincott Williams & Wilkins.

250

CONCEPT

Multiple sclerosis is characterized by periods of remission and exacerbation.

POINTERS

- Factors that can trigger exacerbation of multiple sclerosis:
  Fatigue
  Stress
  Pregnancy
  Acute illness

QUESTION

Which of the following discharge instructions is a priority for the nurse to include in the long range care plan for a client with multiple sclerosis?

1. Referring the client for group therapy
2. Teaching the client to recognize manifestations of myasthenic crisis
3. Monitoring the client for fluctuation of vital signs
4. Teaching the client to identify factors that exacerbate the disease

ANSWER

4

RATIONALE

Inform the client with multiple sclerosis prior to discharge about the factors that may exacerbate the condition, so the client may learn to avoid them.

REFERENCE

Nettina, S. M. (2007). *The Lippincott manual of nursing practice* (8th ed., Philippine ed.). Philadelphia: Lippincott Williams & Wilkins.

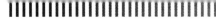

SUBJECT Cerebrovascular Accident (CVA)

CONCEPT
Broca's motor speech area is located in the frontal lobe.

POINTERS

- Cerebrovascular accident is characterized by the sudden loss of brain function resulting from a disruption of blood supply to a part of the brain causing temporary or permanent dysfunction
- Complications of CVA:
  Hemianopsia (loss of vision usually in the vertical half of one or both eyes)
  Emotional lability (mood swings)
  Aphasia (impaired language ability)
  – Receptive/Wernicke's (inability to comprehend)
  – Expressive/Broca's (impaired verbal language expression)
  Dysphagia (difficulty in swallowing)

QUESTION
Which of the following assessment findings indicates the development of a complication in a client with cerebrovascular accident affecting the frontal lobe?

1. Writes short sentences
2. Requests to be turned from side to side every 2 hours
3. Urine output of 60 ml in 2 hours
4. Responds to questions by nodding and shaking the head

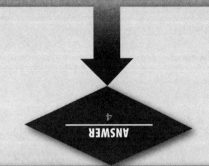

ANSWER
4

RATIONALE
Clients with CVA who nod and shake their head as a way of responding show the presence of expressive aphasia, a manifestation of frontal lobe involvement.

251

NCLEX-RN CATEGORY Reduction of Risk Potential

REFERENCE
Nettina, S. M. (2007). *The Lippincott manual of nursing practice* (8th ed., Philippine ed.). Philadelphia: Lippincott Williams & Wilkins.

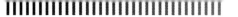

SUBJECT Dysphagia

CONCEPT

Solid foods are easier to swallow than liquids.

QUESTION

Which of the following is an appropriate diet for a client with dysphagia?

1. Mashed potato and orange juice
2. Grapefruit juice and vegetable soup
3. Broiled pork chops and vegetables
4. Milk and creamed soup

POINTERS

Feeding a client with dysphagia

- Instruct the client to eat slowly.
- Place the client in an upright position.
- Administer moist and bolus-shaped foods like scrambled eggs.
- Avoid sticky foods like ice cream, milk, and peanut butter.
- Avoid tepid foods; hot and cold foods are appropriate because it activates the swallowing mechanism.
- For clients with hemiplegia, place the food on the unaffected side of the mouth.

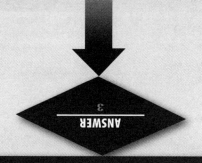

ANSWER

3

RATIONALE

Broiled pork chops and vegetables are solid foods that are easy to swallow for a client with dysphagia.

REFERENCE

Nettina, S. M. (2007). *The Lippincott manual of nursing practice* (8th ed., Philippine ed.). Philadelphia: Lippincott Williams & Wilkins.

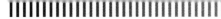

CONCEPT

Retinoblastoma is a genetically transmitted malignant tumor of the retina.

POINTERS

- Retinoblastoma is a congenital tumor of the retina.
- Cat's eye reflex or grayish appearance of the pupil is a common sign.
- Prepare the client for enucleation.
- Refer the parents to a geneticist.

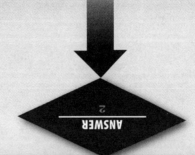

QUESTION

Which of the following clients should be referred to a geneticist?

1. A 3-year-old child with strabismus
2. A 7-year-old boy with grayish discoloration of the pupils
3. A 5-month-old girl with retinal hemorrhage
4. A 10-year-old boy with purulent eye discharge

ANSWER

2

RATIONALE

Grayish discoloration of the pupils (cat's eye reflex) may be associated with retinoblastoma, which is genetically transmitted.

REFERENCE

Nettina, S. M. (2007). *The Lippincott manual of nursing practice* (8th ed., Philippine ed.). Philadelphia: Lippincott Williams & Wilkins.

CONCEPT

Any condition that indicates a complication or is a risk for complication should be reported immediately to the doctor.

POINTERS

Preventing complications after eye surgery

- Avoid activities that will increase intraocular pressure.
- Encourage ambulation.
- Avoid coughing or sneezing.
- Administer medications for pain, nausea, and vomiting as prescribed.

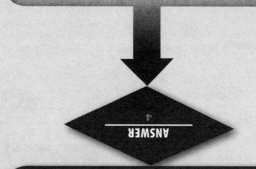

QUESTION

Which finding should the nurse immediately report to the physician on the first postoperative day in a client who had scleral buckling for a detached retina?

1. Ambulating around the bed
2. Listening to music from a radio
3. Maintaining a dependent position
4. Episodes of nausea and vomiting

ANSWER

4

RATIONALE

Episodes of nausea and vomiting may possibly increase intraocular pressure.

REFERENCE

Nettina, S. M. (2007). *The Lippincott manual of nursing practice* (8th ed., Philippine ed.). Philadelphia: Lippincott Williams & Wilkins.

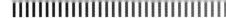

SUBJECT Cataract

CONCEPT
After eye surgery, the client should avoid activities that increase intraocular pressure.

POINTERS
Care of clients with cataracts

- Prepare the client for surgery.
- Postoperatively, instruct the client to avoid activities that require bending, report sudden eye pain (this indicates hemorrhage), and avoid lifting or rapid head movements.

QUESTION
Which of the following activities is/are contraindicated after cataract surgery? Select all that apply.

1. Vacuuming
2. Washing the hair in the bathroom sink
3. Tying shoe laces
4. Cooking
5. Watching TV

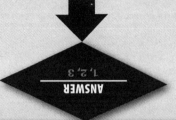

ANSWER
1, 2, 3

RATIONALE
Post-op cataract clients should be advised not to bend from the waist to minimize an increase in intraocular pressure and should be cautioned against coughing or sneezing. Therefore, vacuuming, washing the hair in the bathroom sink, and tying shoe laces are contraindicated.

REFERENCE
Nettina, S. M. (2007). *The Lippincott manual of nursing practice* (8th ed., Philippine ed.). Philadelphia: Lippincott Williams & Wilkins.

CONCEPT

Infectious mononucleosis (the "kissing disease") is caused by the Epstein-Barr virus transmitted through the saliva.

POINTERS

- Infectious mononucleosis is an acute infectious disease of the lymphatic system caused by the Epstein-Barr virus.
- Sore throat is a common symptom.
- Heterophil antibody agglutination test reveals an increase in titer.
- Treatment is symptomatic and supportive.
- Avoid heavy lifting, strenuous exercise, and contact sports until recovery is complete.
- Observe for left upper-quadrant abdominal pain radiating to the left scapula; this indicates splenic rupture.
- The client understood the nurse's health teaching when he/she states, "I will not let others drink from my glass," because the disease is transmitted by saliva and through intimate physical contact like kissing or sharing of utensils.

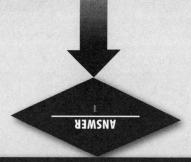

QUESTION

Which of the following personal belongings should not be shared by a client with infectious mononucleosis?

1. A cup
2. A disposable knife
3. Hair spray
4. A belt

ANSWER

RATIONALE

Epstein-Barr virus, the causative agent of infectious mononucleosis, is transmitted through the saliva. Therefore the client's cup should not be shared with others.

REFERENCE

Nettina, S. M. (2007). *The Lippincott manual of nursing practice* (8th ed., Philippine ed.). Philadelphia: Lippincott Williams & Wilkins.

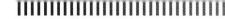
CONCEPT

Cranial nerve VIII, which maintains balance, is affected by acoustic neuroma.

POINTERS

- Acoustic neuroma is a tumor of cranial nerve VIII.
- Tinnitus is a common symptom.
- Caloric stimulation test result indicates no nystagmus.
- Promote safety of the client.
- Keep the client in a supine position if vertigo occurs.

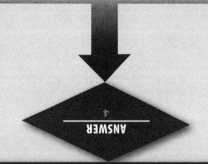

QUESTION

Which of the following nursing diagnoses is the highest priority for a client with acoustic neuroma?

1. Pain
2. Diversional activity deficit
3. Altered tissue perfusion
4. Risk for injury

ANSWER

4

RATIONALE

A client with acoustic neuroma has sensory-perceptual alteration which may result in a fall or injury. Therefore, the priority nursing intervention is to minimize the risk for injury.

NCLEX-RN CATEGORY **Management of Care**

REFERENCE

Nettina, S. M. (2007). *The Lippincott manual of nursing practice* (8th ed., Philippine ed.). Philadelphia: Lippincott Williams & Wilkins.

SUBJECT Osteitis Deformans (Paget's Disease)

CONCEPT

Paget's disease is characterized by deformed bone formation.

POINTERS

- Paget's disease affects men and women.
- It is familial in nature.
- Monitor levels of alkaline phosphatase.
- Commonly treated with alendronate (Fosamax).
- Manifestations:
  - ▸ Joint pain
  - ▸ Chronic headache
  - ▸ Spine curvature
  - ▸ Cartilage damage
  - ▸ Nerve pressure

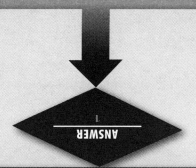

QUESTION

Which of the following nursing diagnoses is appropriate for a client with Paget's disease?

1. Risk for injury
2. Sensory perceptual alteration
3. Altered tissue perfusion
4. Unilateral neglect

ANSWER

1

RATIONALE

Paget's disease is a bone disorder that can lead to osteoarthritis, joint destruction, and bony deformities thereby putting the client at risk for fall or injury.

REFERENCE

Nettina, S. M. (2007). *The Lippincott manual of nursing practice* (8th ed., Philippine ed.). Philadelphia: Lippincott Williams & Wilkins.

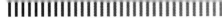

SUBJECT Paget's Disease

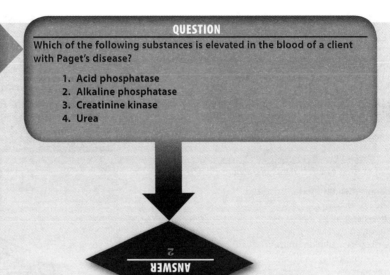

CONCEPT

Alkaline phosphatase is released from destroyed bones in a client with Paget's disease.

QUESTION

Which of the following substances is elevated in the blood of a client with Paget's disease?

1. Acid phosphatase
2. Alkaline phosphatase
3. Creatinine kinase
4. Urea

POINTERS

- Paget's disease of the bone is a skeletal disorder resulting from excessive osteoclastic activity affecting the long bones, pelvis, lumbar vertebrae, and the skull.
- Paget's disease of the nipple is usually associated with underlying intraductal or invasive periareolar eruption.

ANSWER

2

RATIONALE

Serum alkaline phosphatase is usually elevated in Paget's disease. However, serum calcium, phosphorus, and albumin levels remain normal.

259

REFERENCE

Nettina, S. M. (2007). *The Lippincott manual of nursing practice* (8th ed., Philippine ed.). Philadelphia: Lippincott Williams & Wilkins.

NCLEX-RN CATEGORY **Reduction of Risk Potential**

CONCEPT

Skeletal traction is accomplished by ensuring that:

1. Weights are not touching the floor
2. The knot in the rope is not touching the pulley
3. Footplate is not touching the pulley

QUESTION

Which of the following findings in a client in traction interferes with the traction?

1. The ropes and the pulleys are properly aligned
2. The weights are hanging freely
3. The knot in the rope touches the pulley
4. The weights are never removed while the client is repositioned

POINTERS

Principles of nursing care for clients in traction

Trapeze bar overhead is used to raise and lower the upper body
Requires free-hanging weights
Analgesic is given to relieve pain
Check the client's circulation (pulse)
Temperature monitoring
Infection prevention
Output and intake monitoring
Nutrition (appropriate diet)
Skin must be checked frequently

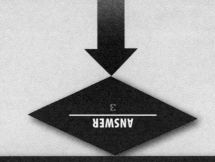

ANSWER
3

RATIONALE

Traction is not accomplished if the knot in the rope is touching the pulley.

NCLEX-RN CATEGORY Basic Care and Comfort

REFERENCE

Nettina, S. M. (2007). *The Lippincott manual of nursing practice* (8th ed., Philippine ed.). Philadelphia: Lippincott Williams & Wilkins.

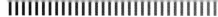

SUBJECT Dunlop's Traction

CONCEPT

Dunlop's traction is used to align fractures of the humerus (horizontal) and to maintain proper alignment of the forearm (vertical).

POINTERS

Dunlop's traction

- Horizontal traction aligns fractures of the humerus.
- Vertical traction maintains proper alignment of forearm.
- Assess for skin breakdown and signs of circulatory impairment and nerve damage.
- Make sure that the weight hangs freely.

QUESTION

Which of the following are the purposes of Dunlop's traction? Select all that apply.

1. To decrease backache
2. To maintain proper alignment of the forearm
3. To align fractures of the humerus
4. To hyperextend the hip and knees

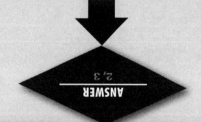

ANSWER
2, 3

RATIONALE

Dunlop's traction is utilized to promote proper alignment of humeral and forearm fractures.

REFERENCE
Nettina, S. M. (2007). *The Lippincott manual of nursing practice* (8th ed., Philippine ed.). Philadelphia: Lippincott Williams & Wilkins.

NCLEX-RN CATEGORY **Basic Care and Comfort**

CONCEPT

Treatment for LCP includes limitation of activities or bed rest.

POINTERS

Common manifestations of Legg-Calvé-Perthes disease

Limping due to synovitis
Contracture deformity
Pain from the knee to the groin

QUESTION

Which of the following nursing diagnoses is appropriate for a client on prolonged bed rest due to Legg-Calvé-Perthes disease?

1. Knowledge deficit
2. Diversional activity deficit
3. Risk for injury
4. Unilateral neglect

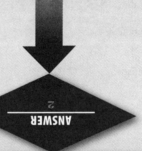

ANSWER

2

RATIONALE

Diversional activity deficit is the appropriate nursing diagnosis for the client being placed on prolonged bed rest. The client may experience boredom due to lack of diversional activities.

REFERENCE

Nettina, S. M. (2007). *The Lippincott manual of nursing practice* (8th ed., Philippine ed.). Philadelphia: Lippincott Williams & Wilkins.

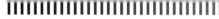

SUBJECT Juvenile Rheumatoid Arthritis (JRA)

CONCEPT

Activities that promote joint mobility are allowed in children with juvenile rheumatoid arthritis.

QUESTION

Which of the following activities is indicated for a client with juvenile rheumatoid arthritis? Select all that apply.

1. Volleyball
2. Swimming
3. Throwing balls
4. Riding a bike

POINTERS

- The goal of care for clients with JRA is to preserve joint function.
- The focus of physical therapy is on strengthening muscles, mobilizing restricted joint motion, and preventing deformities.
- Occupational therapy focus on general mobility and performance of activities of daily living.
- Examples of exercises for children with JRA include kicking a ball, hanging from monkey bars, and stretching.

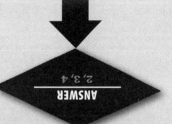

ANSWER
2, 3, 4

RATIONALE

Activities that preserve joint mobility, such as swimming, throwing balls, and riding a bicycle, are allowed in a client with juvenile rheumatoid arthritis.

REFERENCE

Nettina, S. M. (2007). *The Lippincott manual of nursing practice* (8th ed., Philippine ed.). Philadelphia: Lippincott Williams & Wilkins.

CONCEPT

Pemphigus vulgaris is characterized by painful fluid-filled vesicles.

POINTERS

- Pemphigus vulgaris is characterized by the presence of fluid-filled vesicles over 1 cm in size associated with an autoimmune response.
- Manifestations include pain, dysphagia, and lesions on the skin.
- Leukocytosis occurs.
- Administer antibiotics and steroids as ordered.
- Provide potassium permanganate and oatmeal baths.

QUESTION

An appropriate nursing diagnosis for a client with pemphigus vulgaris is which of the following?

1. Altered tissue perfusion
2. Pain
3. Unilateral neglect
4. Altered elimination

ANSWER

2

RATIONALE

Lesions of pemphigus vulgaris gradually enlarge and rupture, forming painful raw and denuded areas that eventually become crusted. Therefore, pain is an appropriate nursing diagnosis.

REFERENCE

Nettina, S. M. (2007). *The Lippincott manual of nursing practice* (8th ed., Philippine ed.). Philadelphia: Lippincott Williams & Wilkins.

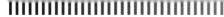

CONCEPT

Accutane is fetotoxic.

POINTERS

- Accutane is an anti-acne medication; it decreases sebaceous gland size.
- It is best taken in the morning with meals because it causes insomnia.
- Female clients should have a pregnancy test as the drug is fetotoxic.
- Ensure that the client is not pregnant.
- Discontinue the drug if visual disturbances occur.

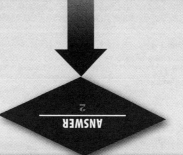

QUESTION

Which of the following discharge instructions should a nurse provide a client who is taking isotretinoin (Accutane)?

1. "Avoid chocolates and fried foods while taking the drug."
2. "Make sure you take your contraceptive pills as prescribed."
3. "It is safe for you to get pregnant."
4. "Abortion is not a potential effect of the drug."

ANSWER

2

RATIONALE

Advise clients to take contraceptive pills while taking accutane to prevent pregnancy because this drug is fetotoxic.

265

REFERENCE

Karch, A. M. (2007). *2008 Lippincott's nursing drug guide*. Philadelphia: Lippincott Williams & Wilkins.

NCLEX-RN CATEGORY **Pharmacological and Parenteral Therapies**

CONCEPT

Scabies is easily transmitted from one person to another.

POINTERS

- Scabies involves infestation with *Sarcoptes scabiei* (itch mite) that occurs through skin or sexual contact.
- Risk factors include overcrowded conditions and poor hygiene.
- Itching that intensifies at night and presence of erythematous nodules or burrows are common signs. These usually appear between fingers, wrists, elbows, axillary folds, waistline, nipples (female), or genitals (male).
- Skin clearing with a therapeutic trial of a pediculicide confirms the diagnosis.
- Apply pediculicide (Kwell) or a scabicide (crotamiton or Eurax) over the entire skin surface.
- Apply topical steroids.
- Practice good handwashing.
- Wear gloves and observe skin precautions for 24 hours after treatment with a pediculicide.
- Instruct the client to apply the lindane lotion from neck down, so that it covers the entire body and their waist for about 15 minutes before dressing. Avoid bathing for 8 to 12 hours.
- Contaminated clothing and linens must be dry cleaned or washed in hot water.
- Do not apply treatment if the skin is inflamed. If allergy to the treatment occurs, wash the skin thoroughly with water.
- Instruct the family members and other close contacts to be treated simultaneously.

QUESTION

The primary goal of care for a hospitalized client with scabies is to:

1. Prevent skin breakdown
2. Prevent transmission to other clients
3. Isolate the client
4. Facilitate early discharge

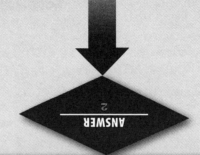

ANSWER

2

RATIONALE

Transmission of scabies occurs through skin or sexual contact. The adult mite can survive without a human host for only 2–3 days.

REFERENCE

Springhouse (Ed.). (2000). *Handbook of infectious diseases.* Philadelphia: Lippincott Williams & Wilkins.

CONCEPT

The best way to prevent drug-induced anaphylaxis is to ask the client if he or she had past drug reactions.

POINTERS

- Common manifestations of anaphylaxis:
  - ▸ Stridor (laryngeal edema)
  - ▸ Lump in the throat
  - ▸ Urticaria
  - ▸ Flushing
  - ▸ Nausea and vomiting

QUESTION

Which of the following interventions should the nurse carry out to prevent anaphylaxis before administering an antibiotic?

1. Check the client's chart for any allergy
2. Ask the client's relatives for history of allergy
3. Ask the client about food idiosyncrasies
4. Ask the client if he had previous reactions to antibiotics

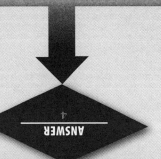

ANSWER

4

RATIONALE

To determine the presence of hypersensitivity reactions to any drug, it is important for the nurse to assess the client's history of previous drug allergies.

REFERENCE

Nettina, S. M. (2007). *The Lippincott manual of nursing practice* (8th ed., Philippine ed.). Philadelphia: Lippincott Williams & Wilkins.

CONCEPT

Bites of pit vipers and coral snakes may lead to neurotoxicity.

POINTERS

Interventions in snake bites

- Immobilize the affected extremity.
- Place the client in recumbent position.
- Administer oxygen, IV fluids, and anti-venom.

QUESTION

Which of the following manifestations is found in clients with rattlesnake bites?

1. Euphoria followed by drowsiness
2. Muscular contraction and rigidity
3. Urticaria with increased sensitivity at the bite site
4. Bleeding and ascites

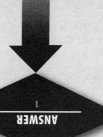

ANSWER

1

RATIONALE

Poisonous snakes like pit vipers (rattlesnakes and copperheads) and coral snakes cause severe envenomation which leads to neurotoxicity. Euphoria followed by dizziness, difficulty swallowing, and paralysis indicate CNS involvement.

REFERENCE

Nettina, S. M. (2007). *The Lippincott manual of nursing practice* (8th ed., Philippine ed.). Philadelphia: Lippincott Williams & Wilkins.

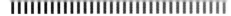

CONCEPT
Lead is usually found in coloring materials.

QUESTION
Who among the following children is most at risk for lead poisoning?

1. A 3-year-old child who lives in a house built in the 1970s
2. A 5-year-old whose father works in a colored glass window factory
3. A 16-year-old who washes his clothes with the washing machine
4. A 10-year-old who is a member of the swimming team

POINTERS
Risk factors

- Lead poisoning is due to consumption by ingestion or inhalation of lead. Risk factors include children who live in houses built before the 1960s (most common), contaminated water, making leaded glass windows, refinishing old furnitures, or folk remedies in some cultures that contain lead, such as Mexican azarcon or greta or Asian paylooah (cure for fever and diarrhea).
- Erythrocyte protoporphyrin level is the initial test. Elevated blood lead level is more than 10 µg/day.
- INTERVENTIONS: Administer the antidote for lead poisoning: Edta and BAL.
- Instruct the parents to eliminate lead hazards at home.
- Monitor level of consciousness (LOC).
- A common complication is iron deficiency anemia.
- Refer the parents to housing authority.

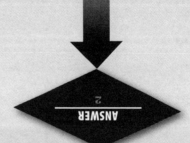

ANSWER
2

RATIONALE
A child whose father works in a leaded glass window factory is at risk for lead poisoning.

REFERENCE
Nettina, S. M. (2007). *The Lippincott manual of nursing practice* (8th ed., Philippine ed.). Philadelphia: Lippincott Williams & Wilkins.

CONCEPT

Children with Down syndrome have a large tongue.

POINTERS

- Down syndrome is characterized by chromosomal abnormality related to an extra chromosome 21 and is usually associated with a congenital heart defect.
- Simian crease, slanting eyes, and large tongue are evident.
- Decreased alpha feto-protein levels are evident.
- Refer the parents for genetic counseling.
- Inform the parents regarding the need for special education.

QUESTION

Which of the following potential problems should the nurse address in the long term care of a child with Down syndrome?

1. Mobility problems
2. Body temperature fluctuation
3. Self-esteem disturbance
4. Feeding problems

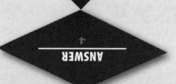

ANSWER

4

RATIONALE

Feeding problems are a potential issue in a child with Down syndrome due to the presence of a large tongue.

REFERENCE

Nettina, S. M. (2007). *The Lippincott manual of nursing practice* (8th ed., Philippine ed.). Philadelphia: Lippincott Williams & Wilkins.

SUBJECT Fetal Alcohol Syndrome (FAS)

CONCEPT

Fetal alcohol syndrome is characterized by difficulty in sucking.

POINTERS

- FAS occurs when there is direct ethanol toxicity to a developing fetus.
- Manifestations include dyspnea, increased muscle tone, tremulousness, lethargy, poor sucking reflex, facial abnormalities, and seizure.
- Administer Valium as prescribed.
- Decrease environmental stimuli.
- Provide small frequent feedings.
- Have resuscitative equipment available.

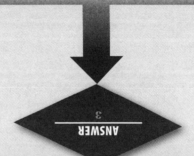

QUESTION

Which of the following statements, if made by a one week postpartum client, reflects a need for further evaluation of her baby?

1. "My baby sleeps most of the day."
2. "My baby's feet and hands are bluish."
3. "My baby always falls asleep after a minute of sucking."
4. "My baby seems to be losing weight."

ANSWER

3

RATIONALE

A baby that falls asleep after a minute of sucking indicates difficulty in sucking, a characteristic of neonates with fetal alcohol syndrome.

271

REFERENCE
Nettina, S. M. (2007). *The Lippincott manual of nursing practice* (8th ed., Philippine ed.). Philadelphia: Lippincott Williams & Wilkins.

NCLEX-RN CATEGORY Reduction of Risk Potential

NCLEX-RN CATEGORY Health Promotion and Maintenance

CONCEPT

West Nile virus is transmitted by the bite of infected mosquito.

POINTERS

- West Nile virus causes inflammation of the brain.
- It is transmitted to humans by the bite of a mosquito.
- Birds serve as the reservoir of the West Nile virus.
- Mosquitoes serve as the vectors.
- The incubation period is from 5 to 15 days.
- Apply insect repellent on the skin like DEET (N,N-diethyl-*meta*-toluamide).
- Early manifestations include fever, headache, and body malaise.

QUESTION

Which of the following instructions will help prevent infection with West Nile virus?

1. Avoid exposure to deer ticks
2. Eliminate mosquito breeding places
3. Use sunscreen lotion when outdoors
4. Avoid going barefoot at home

ANSWER

2

RATIONALE

The West Nile virus is transmitted to humans by the bite of a mosquito (primarily Culex species) infected with the virus. Eliminating mosquito breeding places will reduce the risk of becoming infected.

REFERENCE

Springhouse (Ed.). (2000). *Handbook of infectious diseases.* Philadelphia: Lippincott Williams & Wilkins.

CONCEPT

Rotavirus infection is manifested by acute gastroenteritis

POINTERS

- Rotavirus is the most common cause of severe diarrhea among children.
- Rotavirus gastroenteritis usually starts with a fever, nausea, and vomiting followed by diarrhea.
- PRIORITY: Oral rehydration

QUESTION

A client with rotavirus infection should be placed under what type of isolation precautions?

1. Contact
2. Droplet
3. Airborne
4. Standard

ANSWER

1

RATIONALE

The primary mode of transmission of rotavirus is fecal-oral, although some have reported low titers of virus in respiratory tract secretions and other bodily fluids. Due to the instability of the virus, transmission can occur through ingestion of contaminated water or food and contact with contaminated surfaces. The client should therefore be placed in contact isolation precautions.

REFERENCE

Springhouse (Ed.). (2000). *Handbook of infectious diseases.* Philadelphia: Lippincott Williams & Wilkins.

273

NCLEX-RN CATEGORY Safety and Infection Control

CONCEPT

Uncooked meat is a potential source of toxoplasmosis.

POINTERS

- Fecal-oral contamination from infected cats transmits toxoplasmosis.
- Cooking, drying, heating, or freezing destroys the cysts that cause toxoplasmosis.
- Treatment involves administration of sulfonamides and pyrimethamine.

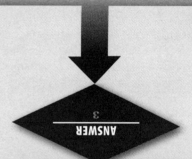

QUESTION

Which of the following instructions should the nurse give to a client who is at risk for toxoplasmosis?

1. "Wash your dishes in a diluted bleach solution."
2. "Wear gloves when preparing your meals."
3. "Avoid eating uncooked meat."
4. "Avoid crowded areas."

ANSWER

3

RATIONALE

Ingestion of tissue cysts in raw or undercooked meat or fecal-oral contamination from infected cats transmits toxoplasmosis

REFERENCE

Springhouse (Ed.). (2000). *Handbook of infectious diseases*. Philadelphia: Lippincott Williams & Wilkins.

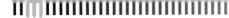

SUBJECT Lyme Disease

CONCEPT

Lyme disease is usually transmitted through the bite of black legged ticks initially found in Lyme, Connecticut.

POINTERS

- Lyme disease is a multi-system infectious syndrome commonly affecting the skin, nervous system, heart, and joints.
- It is characterized by a bull's eye rash usually found in moist parts of the body, usually described as "rounded rings" of rash.
- Ascertain if the client was exposed to deer ticks.
- Instruct the client to wear light colored clothing when going to the forest/woods or have himself/herself vaccinated.
- When bitten by a tick, remove it by exerting a slow, steady, upward pull and avoid squeezing it.

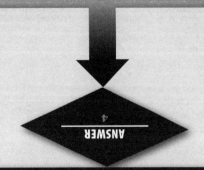

QUESTION

Who among the following clients is most at risk for Lyme disease?

1. A 15-year-old adolescent from New York
2. A 20-year-old pregnant client from California
3. A 40-year-old obese client from New Mexico
4. A 30-year-old male from Connecticut

ANSWER

4

RATIONALE

A person from Connecticut is at high risk for Lyme disease because the ticks causing the disease were initially found in that area.

REFERENCE

Nettina, S. M. (2007). *The Lippincott manual of nursing practice* (8th ed., Philippine ed.). Philadelphia: Lippincott Williams & Wilkins.

SUBJECT Fifth's Disease

CONCEPT

Fifth's disease is transmitted via respiratory secretion.

276

POINTERS

- Fifth's disease is infection caused by human parvo virus B19.
- It is transmitted via respiratory secretion.
- Common among children between 4–12 years old
- Resolves in about 7–10 days
- Usual manifestations include a red rash on cheeks (slapped cheek appearance), low grade fever, malaise, joint pain, and swelling in the hands, wrists, and knees.

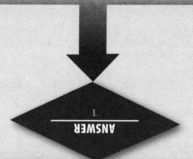

QUESTION

Which instructions should the nurse emphasize when providing discharge teaching to a client with Fifth's disease?

1. "Cover your mouth and nose when coughing and sneezing."
2. "Separate your towels from the rest of the family."
3. "Avoid having a tattoo."
4. "Avoid contact with pet dogs."

ANSWER

1

RATIONALE

Fifth's disease is transmitted via respiratory secretions, therefore the client should be instructed to cover the mouth and nose when coughing and sneezing to prevent the spread of infection.

REFERENCE

Gapuz, R. *The ABCs of passing foreign nursing exams.* Philippines: Gapuz Publications.

NCLEX-RN CATEGORY Safety and Infection Control

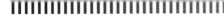

CONCEPT

Carpal tunnel syndrome is associated with job-related tasks involving the wrist.

QUESTION

Carpal tunnel syndrome is usually associated with which of the following jobs? Select all that apply.

1. Typists
2. Computer operators
3. Assembly line workers
4. Truck drivers
5. Carpenters
6. Cheerleaders
7. Singers

POINTERS

- Carpal tunnel syndrome most commonly occurs in women aged 30–50 years old.
- Causes include rheumatoid arthritis, diabetes mellitus, hypothyroidism, acromegaly, amyloidosis, and pregnancy (producing edema in the carpal tunnel).

ANSWER

1, 2, 3, 4, 5

RATIONALE

Activities or jobs that require repetitive flexion and extension of the wrist (e.g., keyboard use) may pose an occupational risk. Often no underlying cause is found.

REFERENCE

Nettina, S. M. (2007). *The Lippincott manual of nursing practice* (8th ed., Philippine ed.). Philadelphia: Lippincott Williams & Wilkins.

NCLEX-RN CATEGORY Reduction of Risk Potential

CONCEPT

Pilocarpine is used in clients with Sjögren's syndrome to improve salivation.

POINTERS

- Sjögren's syndrome is a chronic, inflammatory autoimmune process that affects the lacrimal and salivary glands
- Common manifestations:
  - ▸ Keratoconjunctivitis
  - ▸ Xerostomia (dry mouth)
  - ▸ Xerodermia (dry skin)
  - ▸ Dyspareunia

QUESTION

Which of the following medications is given to clients with Sjögren's syndrome to improve salivation?

1. Atropine sulfate
2. Cyclophosphamide (Cytoxan)
3. Pilocarpine
4. Furosemide (Lasix)

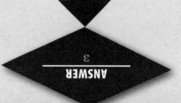

ANSWER

3

RATIONALE

Pilocarpine is a cholinergic drug given orally to improve salivation in clients with Sjögren's syndrome.

REFERENCE

Nettina, S. M. (2007). *The Lippincott manual of nursing practice* (8th ed., Philippine ed.). Philadelphia: Lippincott Williams & Wilkins.

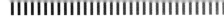

CONCEPT

The priority for a client with delirium tremens is to maintain physiologic integrity.

POINTERS

- Delirium tremens usually occurs 2–4 days after a client's last alcohol intake. It is due to faulty metabolism of alcohol.
- Increased vital signs and coarse hand tremors occur.
- Blood alcohol level is more than 0.2%.
- Provide a well-lighted room for the client because they fear shadows.
- Instruct the client to abstain from alcohol.
- Administer chlordiazepoxide (Librium) to the client; it is considered the drug of choice for acute alcohol withdrawal syndrome.

QUESTION

Which of the following nursing interventions is a priority for a client with delirium tremens?

1. Maintaining psychosocial integrity
2. Promotion of optimum level of functioning
3. Maintaining physiological integrity
4. Providing a consistent routine

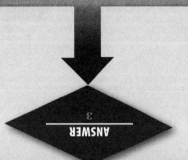

ANSWER 3

RATIONALE

Maintaining physiological integrity is the top priority nursing intervention for clients with delirium tremens.

279

REFERENCE

Nettina, S. M. (2007). *The Lippincott manual of nursing practice* (8th ed., Philippine ed.). Philadelphia: Lippincott Williams & Wilkins.

NCLEX-RN CATEGORY Management of Care

CONCEPT

Denial is the reaction of a client to unacceptable situations.

POINTERS

- Denial is the refusal to admit an unacceptable idea or behavior.
- The nurse should recognize that denial is the client's normal reaction to stressful events.
- Denial is a common problem among alcoholic clients.

QUESTION

Which of the following statements, if made by a woman who delivers a child with a cleft palate, indicates a denial response of clients to such situations?

1. "This is heaven's curse."
2. "What will other people say?"
3. "Are you sure you brought me my baby?"
4. "Things like this really happen, it's nobody's fault."

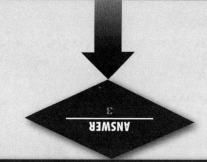

ANSWER

3

RATIONALE

The statement "Are you sure you brought me my baby?" is an example of denial whereby the mother initially could not accept the baby's condition.

REFERENCE

Nettina, S. M. (2007). *The Lippincott manual of nursing practice* (8th ed., Philippine ed.). Philadelphia: Lippincott Williams & Wilkins.

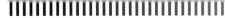

CONCEPT

Buspar takes 1 to 2 weeks to achieve the desired anti-anxiety effect.

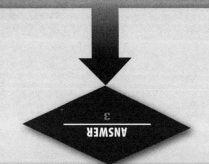

QUESTION

In a client taking buspirone (Buspar), the nurse should evaluate for the therapeutic effects at which of the following times?

1. Immediately after administering the drug
2. Within 6 months of taking the drug
3. In 1 to 2 weeks after taking the drug
4. After all the prescribed dose of the drug has been consumed

ANSWER

3

POINTERS

Evidence of therapeutic effects of certain drugs:

- Heparin: 1–2 days
- Coumadin: 2–5 days
- Antiparkinsonian: 1–3 days
- Lithium: 7–10 days
- Allopurinol: 1–3 weeks
- TCAs: 2–4 weeks
- Iron: 2–4 weeks
- Thyroid agents: 2–4 weeks

RATIONALE

It will take up to 2 weeks for the drug to achieve full therapeutic effect, in which a noticeable change in the client's behavior can be seen.

REFERENCE

Karch, A. M. (2007). *2008 Lippincott's nursing drug guide*. Philadelphia: Lippincott Williams & Wilkins.

281

NCLEX-RN CATEGORY **Pharmacological and Parenteral Therapies**

CONCEPT

Depressed clients usually experience problems in sleep, bowel elimination, and lack of energy.

POINTERS

- Depression is characterized by a mood state of gloom.
- Signs and symptoms include:
  Depressed mood
  Energy loss
  Psychomotor agitation
  Recurrent thoughts of death and suicide
  Excessive or diminished sleep
  Significant weight gain or weight loss
  Significant distress or impairment in social functioning
  Excessive or inappropriate guilt
  Diminished interest or pleasure (anhedonia)
- Adapt a kind but firm attitude when dealing with the client.
- Inform the client that it takes 2–3 weeks before the therapeutic effects of antidepressant drugs become evident.
- Provide monotonous and repetitive activities to the client.
- Implement suicide precautions at the onset of depression and when depression begins to lessen or abate.

QUESTION

Which of the following manifestations are found in a client with depression? Select all that apply.

1. Insomnia
2. Anesthesia of body parts
3. Hard stools
4. Agnosia
5. Fatigue

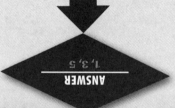

ANSWER 1, 3, 5

RATIONALE

Depression is characterized by depressed mood or decreased interest or pleasure in all or almost all activities. Typical symptoms include headache, sleep disturbances, chronic fatigue, chest pain, nausea, vomiting, constipation, weight loss or gain, urinary retention, slouched posture, decreased mood and activity, restlessness, amenorrhea, impotence, and decreased libido.

REFERENCE
Keltner, N. L, Bostrom, C. E., & Schweke, L. H. (2006). *Psychiatric nursing* (5th ed.). Philadelphia: Mosby.

CONCEPT

Preserved foods usually contain tyramine.

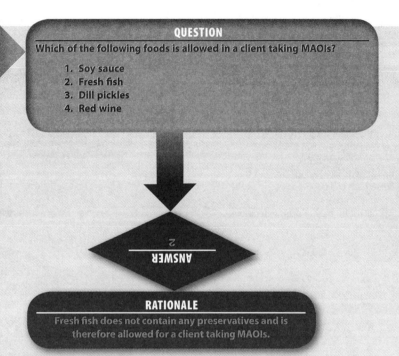

QUESTION

Which of the following foods is allowed in a client taking MAOIs?

1. Soy sauce
2. Fresh fish
3. Dill pickles
4. Red wine

ANSWER

2

RATIONALE

Fresh fish does not contain any preservatives and is therefore allowed for a client taking MAOIs.

POINTERS

- MAOIs increase appetite and promote adequate sleep.
- They are best taken after meals.
- Report headache as it indicates a hypertensive crisis.
- Avoid tyramine-containing foods like:
  Avocado
  Banana
  Cheddar and aged cheese
  Soysauce and preserved foods
- Monitor the client's BP.

283

REFERENCE
Gapuz, R. *The ABCs of passing foreign nursing exams.* Philippines: Gapuz Publications.

NCLEX-RN CATEGORY **Pharmacological and Parenteral Therapies**

284

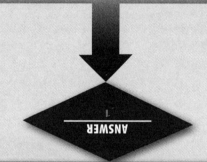

CONCEPT

Dysthymic disorder is characterized by depressed mood that occurs over a two-year period.

POINTERS

- To bolster the client's self esteem, accept them as they are.
- Point out every small visible accomplishment, like saying "I'm glad that you took a bath today."
- Spend time with client.
- Assist the client in making simple decisions.

QUESTION

Which of the following interventions is the priority for a client with dysthymic disorder?

1. Assess for current suicide risk
2. Administer antidepressants as ordered
3. Remain with the client during mealtimes
4. Collaborate with occupational and physical therapists to determine the client's functional abilities

ANSWER

1

RATIONALE

A client with dysthymic disorder is at high risk for committing suicide. Therefore, the nurse should assess the client regularly for suicide risk.

REFERENCE

Keltner, N. L., Bostrom, C. E., & Schweke, L. H. (2006). *Psychiatric nursing* (5th ed.). Philadelphia: Mosby.

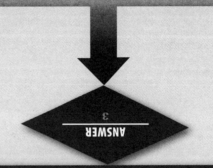

CONCEPT

Elderly clients with chronic illness are usually successful on their first suicidal attempt.

POINTERS

Suicidal risk factors

Sex: more women attempt suicide; more men commit suicide
Unsuccessful previous attempts
Identification with a family member who committed suicide
Chronic
Illness
Depression
Age: between 18–25 and above 40 years
Loss of a loved one

QUESTION

Which of the following clients is at greatest risk for suicide?

1. A 16-year-old male adolescent with history of drug addiction
2. A 40-year-old divorced female with midlife crisis
3. A 68-year-old female with multiple sclerosis who recently lost her husband in a car accident
4. A 35-year-old with bipolar disorder

ANSWER
3

RATIONALE

Early loss, decreased social support, chronic illness, or recent divorce are among the risk factors for suicide. Therefore, a 68-year-old female client with multiple sclerosis who recently lost her husband is at greater risk for committing suicide.

REFERENCE
Nettina, S. M. (2007). *The Lippincott manual of nursing practice* (8th ed., Philippine ed.). Philadelphia: Lippincott Williams & Wilkins.

CONCEPT

An increase in appetite and adequate sleep are indicators of effectiveness of antidepressants.

POINTERS

- Antidepressants should not be given with citrus juices as these may decrease absorption.
- It usually takes 2–3 weeks before initial therapeutic effects become evident and 3–4 weeks for the full therapeutic effects.
- Once the client shows improvement, assess the client for signs of suicide.

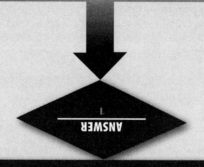

QUESTION

Which of the following client's behaviors indicates that the antidepressants are effective?

1. The client asks for a snack from the nurse
2. The client sleeps 12 hours a day
3. The client's blood pressure decreases
4. The client's mood remains the same

ANSWER

1

RATIONALE

Improvement in the client's appetite as shown by the client's desire for a snack indicates a positive response to the antidepressant medications.

REFERENCE

Karch, A. M. (2007). *2008 Lippincott's nursing drug guide*. Philadelphia: Lippincott Williams & Wilkins.

CONCEPT

According to Maslow's hierarchy of needs, the need for food is among the most important.

QUESTION

Which of the following interventions is the nursing priority when providing care for a client with catatonic schizophrenia?

1. Assist the client with bathing
2. Stay with the client at all times to show reassurance
3. Interact with the client at regular intervals
4. Assist the client with feeding

POINTERS

- Catatonic schizophrenia is characterized by a marked disturbance in motor function.
- Clients may need careful supervision to prevent them from hurting themselves or others.
- Associated problems include malnutrition, exhaustion, hyperpyrexia, or self-inflicted injury.

ANSWER

4

RATIONALE

Using Maslow's hierarchy of needs theory to prioritize, the client's physiological needs come first. Food is a physiological need and is a nursing priority.

REFERENCE

Sadock, B. J., & Sadock, V. A. (2007). *Kaplan and Sadock's synopsis of psychiatry* (10th ed.). Philadelphia: Lippincott Williams & Wilkins.

CONCEPT

Clozaril causes leukopenia.

POINTERS

- Clozaril decreases the symptoms of schizophrenia.
- It is best taken after meals.
- Inform the client about a weekly blood check for WBCs.
- Report fever, sore throat, lethargy, malaise, or signs of infection.
- Smoking may decrease drug effectiveness.
- Rise slowly to avoid dizziness.
- Ice chips or sugarless gum may help relieve dry mouth.
- If the client's WBC count drops below 3,500/mm³, monitor the client for signs of infection.
- If the client's WBC count drops below 2,000/mm³, place the client in protective isolation.
- Avoid the use of St. John's wort while taking Clozaril as it may decrease Clozaril levels.
- Monitor RR; Clozaril may cause respiratory arrest.

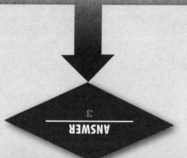

QUESTION

Which of the following actions constitute an act of negligence on the part of the nurse?

1. Administering Clozaril to a client after meals
2. Instructing the client on Clozaril to suck on ice chips
3. Administering Clozaril to a client despite a WBC count of 1,500/mm³
4. Withholding Clozaril to a client who uses St. John's wort

ANSWER

3

RATIONALE

Clozaril decreases WBC count, therefore administration of the drug in a client with a low WBC count of 1,500/mm³ is a negligent act.

REFERENCE

Karch, A. M. (2007). *2008 Lippincott's nursing drug guide*. Philadelphia: Lippincott Williams & Wilkins.

SUBJECT Anorexia Nervosa

CONCEPT

Parents of anorexic clients are often domineering or perfectionists.

POINTERS

- Anorexia nervosa is characterized by fear of gaining weight.
- Amenorrhea (absence of menses for at least three consecutive months) in the absence of other organic causes is a common symptom. Other signs and symptoms are:

  Amenorrhea

  No other organic factor accounts for the weight loss

  Obviously thin but feels fat

  Refusal to maintain ideal body weight

  Epigastric discomforts

  X - symptoms like hiding foods and collecting recipes

  Intense fear of gaining weight

  Always thinking about food

- Decreased K levels due to vomiting and hypoglycemia
- Monitor the client's weight.
- Institute family therapy since many parents of anorexics are rigid, perfectionists, and domineering.

QUESTION

The mother of a teenage girl makes all of the following statements. Which one needs further exploration by the nurse?

1. "I'll bring my daughter to the dermatologist for acne treatment."
2. "I make it a point to check on her every now and then."
3. "Girls sometimes just want to have fun."
4. "I asked her to tell me if she needs anything."

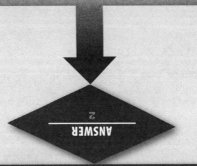

ANSWER

2

RATIONALE

Statement two reflects a tendency of the mother to be rigid and dominating. This is a common characteristic of parents of anorexic teenagers.

REFERENCE

Nettina, S. M. (2007). *The Lippincott manual of nursing practice* (8th ed., Philippine ed.). Philadelphia. Lippincott Williams & Wilkins.

CONCEPT

Bulimic clients usually induce vomiting after meals.

POINTERS

- Bulimia involves binge eating and purging.
- Weight loss is a common sign. Other signs and symptoms include:

  Binge eating

  Under strict dieting or vigorous exercise

  Lack of control over eating binges

  Induced vomiting

  Minimum of two binge eating episodes in a week for a period of three months

  Increased or persistent concern over body size or shape

  Abuse of laxatives or diuretics

- Hypokalemia and hypoglycemia occur.
- Monitor the client's weight.
- Stay with the client for at least 30 minutes to 1 hour after meals.

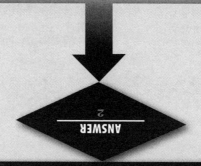

QUESTION

Which of the following behaviors of a client with bulimia nervosa reflects a need for further investigation?

1. The client attends a support group gathering
2. The client uses the bathroom immediately after meals
3. The client stays in the dayroom after meals
4. The client recognizes the presence of a problem

ANSWER

2

RATIONALE

A bulimic client who uses the bathroom immediately after meals should be investigated further given that bulimic clients induce vomiting after binge eating.

REFERENCE

Nettina, S. M. (2007). *The Lippincott manual of nursing practice* (8th ed., Philippine ed.). Philadelphia: Lippincott Williams & Wilkins.

CONCEPT

Hypokalemia occurs in bulimia.

POINTERS

Complications of bulimia nervosa

Cardiac dysrhythmias
Hypokalemia
Obesity
Metabolic acidosis
Esophageal tear
Dental erosion

PRIORITY: Nutrition planning to accomplish weight goal

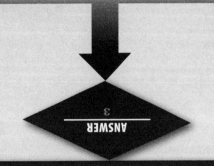

QUESTION

Which of the following laboratory test findings supports a diagnosis of bulimia nervosa?

1. Calcium level of 9.5 mg/dl
2. Blood sugar level of 160 mg/dl
3. Potassium level of 2.6 mEq/L
4. Potassium level of 6.3 mEq/L

ANSWER

3

RATIONALE

Induced vomiting that occurs in a bulimic client may result in electrolyte imbalances such as hypokalemia, hyponatremia, hypochloremia, or elevated bicarbonate. The normal serum potassium level is 3.5 to 5 mEq/L.

291

REFERENCE
Nettina, S. M. (2007). *The Lippincott manual of nursing practice* (8th ed., Philippine ed.). Philadelphia: Lippincott Williams & Wilkins.

NCLEX-RN CATEGORY **Reduction of Risk Potential**

SUBJECT Fluvoxamine Maleate (Luvox)

CONCEPT

Luvox is used to treat obsessive-compulsive disorder.

POINTERS

- Luvox is a selective serotonin reuptake inhibitor (SSRI).
- It is best taken at bedtime.
- Common side effects include dizziness, drowsiness, insomnia, and reversible sexual dysfunction.
- Report the presence of rash, mania, seizures, and severe weight loss to the physician.

QUESTION

Which of the following behaviors, if found in a client with obsessive-compulsive disorder, is indicative of the effectiveness of fluvoxamine maleate (Luvox)?

1. Decreased episodes of hallucination
2. Stability of mood
3. Decreased incidence of violent behavior
4. Decreased time for performing their rituals

ANSWER

4

RATIONALE

Luvox decreases the ritualistic behavior of a client with obsessive-compulsive disorder.

REFERENCE

Karch, A. M. (2007). *2008 Lippincott's nursing drug guide*. Philadelphia: Lippincott Williams & Wilkins.

CONCEPT

Attend to the client's physiologic needs first.

QUESTION

Which of the following data entered in a manic client's chart should the nurse first pay particular attention to?

1. The client promises to buy clothes for all her fellow clients
2. The client verbalizes that her self-esteem is threatened
3. The client verbalizes feeling depressed sometimes
4. The client has not slept for 36 hours

ANSWER

4

RATIONALE

The need for sleep is the primary consideration of the nurse because it is a physiologic need.

POINTERS

Maslow's hierarchy of needs

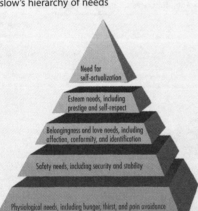

Need for self-actualization

Esteem needs, including prestige and self-respect

Belongingness and love needs, including affection, conformity, and identification

Safety needs, including security and stability

Physiological needs, including hunger, thirst, and pain avoidance

293

REFERENCE

Keltner, N. L., Bostrom, C. E., & Schweke, L. H. (2006). *Psychiatric nursing* (5th ed.). Philadelphia: Mosby.

NCLEX-RN CATEGORY **Psychosocial Integrity**

SUBJECT Depakene (Valproic Acid)

CONCEPT

Depakene irritates the oral mucosa, so it should not be crushed.

POINTERS

Drugs that should not be crushed
- Accutane (irritant)
- Azulfidine (enteric coated)
- Depakene (irritates the mouth)
- Ecotrin
- Indocin
- Mestinon timespans
- MS contin
- Nexium
- Noctec
- Ritalin
- Wellbutrin

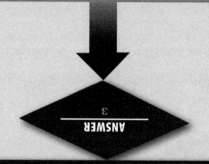

QUESTION

Which of the following actions of the LPN (licensed practical nurse) needs to be corrected by the RN (registered nurse)?

1. Administering Fosamax with water
2. Giving Ritalin in the morning after breakfast
3. Crushing Depakene before giving it
4. Withholding Wellbutrin in a client with seizure episode

ANSWER

3

RATIONALE

Depakene should not be crushed because it irritates the oral mucosa.

REFERENCE

Karch, A. M. (2007). *2008 Lippincott's nursing drug guide*. Philadelphia: Lippincott Williams & Wilkins.

CONCEPT

Clients with dissociative identity disorder are often suicidal.

POINTERS

Clinical manifestations of dissociative identity disorder
- Dissociative identity disorder is characterized by the presence of two or more identities or personalities that take control of a person's behavior.
- The priority goal of care for clients with the disorder is to integrate the personalities with the original personality.
- The nurse should also establish a contract to reduce self-harm and violence.

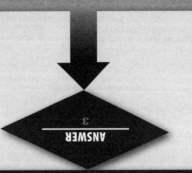

QUESTION

Which of the following nursing diagnoses is the highest priority for a client with dissociative identity disorder?

1. Sensory perceptual alteration
2. Diversional activity deficit
3. Risk for self-directed violence
4. Altered thought process

ANSWER

3

RATIONALE

Clients with dissociative identity disorder may develop aggressive behavior toward themselves or others and such behavior may include suicide attempts or self-mutilation.

REFERENCE

Nettina, S. M. (2007). *The Lippincott manual of nursing practice* (8th ed., Philippine ed.). Philadelphia: Lippincott Williams & Wilkins.

SUBJECT Delirium Tremens

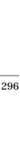
CONCEPT

The onset of delirium tremens is 12 hours to 1 week after the client's last drink.

POINTERS

- Delirium tremens usually occur 2–4 days after a client's last alcohol intake. It is due to faulty metabolism of alcohol.
- It is characterized by a blood alcohol level of more than 0.2%.
- Provide a well-lighted room for the client because they fear shadows.
- Instruct the client to abstain from alcohol.
- Administer chlordiazepoxide (Librium) to the client; it is considered as the drug of choice for acute alcohol withdrawal syndrome.

QUESTION

A client with alcohol abuse is admitted to the detoxification unit. Which of the following questions should the nurse ask the client immediately?

1. "Are you having problems with your husband?"
2. "At what age did you start drinking?"
3. "What did you eat in the last 24 hours?"
4. "When was your last drink?"

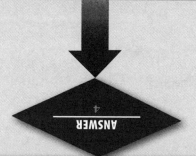

ANSWER

4

RATIONALE

Delirium tremens occur 12 hours to 1 week after a client's last intake of alcohol. Therefore, during the initial assessment the nurse should ask the client when the client's last alcohol intake was to determine its probable recognition and intervention.

REFERENCE

Keltner, N. L., Bostrom, C. E., & Schweke, L. H. (2006). *Psychiatric nursing* (5th ed.). Philadelphia: Mosby.

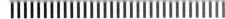

CONCEPT

Loss of central vision occurs in age-related macular degeneration.

POINTERS

- AMD is an age-related eye disorder characterized by bilateral loss of central vision with preservation of some peripheral vision.
- It comes in two forms:
  ▸ Atrophic or dry form
  ▸ Exudative or wet form
- There is no treatment.
- It is progressive.

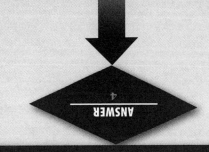

QUESTION

Which of the following manifestations occur in age-related macular degeneration (AMD)?

1. Floating spots in the eyes
2. Watery eyes
3. Loss of peripheral vision
4. Loss of central vision

ANSWER

4

RATIONALE

Loss of central vision is indicative of age-related macular degeneration.

REFERENCE

Nettina, S. M. (2007). *The Lippincott manual of nursing practice* (8th ed., Philippine ed.). Philadelphia: Lippincott Williams & Wilkins.

CONCEPT

Xerostomia or dry mouth occurs with aging.

POINTERS

Common changes in the elderly:
- Decreased visual acuity
- Decreased hearing ability
- Increased sensitivity to glare
- Decreased tolerance to narcotics
- Increased reaction time
- Difficulty in differentiating blue and green colors
- Taste buds are lost from front to the back (sweet and salty tastes are lost first, bitter and sour taste remain longer).

QUESTION

Which of the following statements indicates an expected change in the elderly?

1. "I drink fluids while eating because my mouth feels dry."
2. "I don't drive at night because I see floating spots."
3. "I put on less perfume because I can strongly smell it."
4. "I use less salt for my food because I have heightened taste."

ANSWER

1

RATIONALE

The client's statement "I drink fluids while eating because my mouth feels dry" is indicative of xerostomia, which is a common problem among elderly people.

REFERENCE

Nettina, S. M. (2007). *The Lippincott manual of nursing practice* (8th ed., Philippine ed.). Philadelphia: Lippincott Williams & Wilkins.

CONCEPT

Xerosis is characterized by dry, irritated skin.

POINTERS

Skin care for the elderly

- Avoid excessive use of soap
- Avoid direct application of heat and cold
- Encourage use of sunscreen during all outdoor activities
- Increase fluid intake

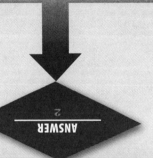

QUESTION

Which of the following interventions is appropriate for an elderly client with xerosis?

1. Immerse the body in cold water for 30 minutes
2. Increase fluid intake to 2,000 ml daily
3. Use alcohol on the skin
4. Use soap at least 5 times a day

ANSWER

2

RATIONALE

Xerosis is a common problem in the elderly. Treatment should include drinking 2,000 ml of liquid daily.

299

NCLEX-RN CATEGORY Health Promotion and Maintenance

REFERENCE

Nettina, S. M. (2007). *The Lippincott manual of nursing practice* (8th ed., Philippine ed.). Philadelphia: Lippincott Williams & Wilkins.

300

CONCEPT

Inflammatory response in the elderly is delayed.

POINTERS

Early signs of infection in the elderly include:

Increasing pain
Fatigue
Anorexia
Mental status changes

QUESTION

Which of the following are early indicators of infection in the elderly? Select all that apply.

1. Fever
2. Redness
3. Fatigue
4. Swelling
5. Anorexia

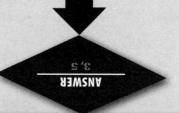

ANSWER
3, 5

RATIONALE

The older person may be unable to respond to an illness. These altered responses reinforce the need for the nurse to monitor older clients closely and be alert to signs of impending systemic complications. Fatigue and anorexia are two of the early signs of infection in the elderly.

REFERENCE

Smeltzer, S. C., Bare, B. G., Hinkle, J. L., & Cheever, K. H. (2006). *Brunner and Suddarth's textbook of medical-surgical nursing.* Philadelphia: Lippincott Williams & Wilkins.

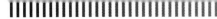

SUBJECT Therapeutic Levels of Certain Drugs

CONCEPT

Drugs with narrow therapeutic range require serum level monitoring.

POINTERS

Drugs with narrow therapeutic range

Lithium
- Acute dose: 0.5–1.5 mEq/L
- Maintenance dose: 0.5–1.2 mEq/L
- For elderly: 0.4–0.8 mEq/L

Theophylline
- 10–20 ug/dL

Dilantin
- 10–20 ug/dL

Haldol
- 6 mg/day in the elderly

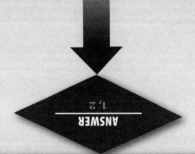

QUESTION

Which of the following drugs will require regular monitoring of plasma levels? Select all that apply.

1. Lithium (Eskalith)
2. Theophylline (Theo-Dur)
3. Aspirin
4. Imipramine (Tofranil)

ANSWER

1, 2

RATIONALE

Lithium and theophylline are drugs with a narrow therapeutic range that are close to toxic levels. Therefore, requiring frequent serum level monitoring is necessary.

301

REFERENCE

Karch, A. M. (2007). *2008 Lippincott's nursing drug guide.* Philadelphia: Lippincott Williams & Wilkins.

NCLEX-RN CATEGORY **Pharmacological and Parenteral Therapies**

CONCEPT

A consistent, familiar, and safe environment is best to promote function of the elderly.

POINTERS

Normal changes of aging

- Decreased dark adaptation
- Difficulty in differentiating blue and green
- Needs louder sound to stimulate hearing
- Decreased appetite
- Has a tendency to lean forward

Safety considerations

- Provide sufficient glare-free lights
- Elevated toilet seats
- Provide skid proof mats in the shower

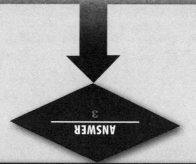

QUESTION

When conducting a home visit to the house of an elderly client, which of the following observations should the nurse address first?

1. Loud volume of the television set
2. Wall to wall carpet in the living room
3. New placement of furniture
4. Use of indirect lighting

ANSWER

3

RATIONALE

Furniture should remain unchanged because elderly clients function best in familiar settings.

REFERENCE

Nettina, S. M. (2007). *The Lippincott manual of nursing practice* (8th ed., Philippine ed.). Philadelphia: Lippincott Williams & Wilkins.

CONCEPT

The risk factors for osteoporosis include:
- Aging
- Immobility
- Menopause
- Smoking and long term use of steroids

POINTERS

- Osteoporosis is the loss of bone matrix leading to bone weakness making it susceptible to fracture. It is usually associated with smoking, menopause, immobility, and hyperparathyroidism.
- X-ray reveals osteoporosis.
- Increase calcium and vitamin D in the diet.
- Use of conjugated estrogen therapy for menopausal women. Avoid smoking.
- Encourage the client to perform active-weight bearing exercises like brisk walking, jumping rope, hiking, tennis, and ballroom dancing.
- Swimming does not meet the criteria for resistance needed to prevent osteoporosis.

QUESTION

Which of the following assessment findings is indicative of a complication from a long-term steroid therapy?

1. Weight gain
2. Increased appetite
3. Gradual decrease in height
4. Insomnia

ANSWER

3

RATIONALE

Steroids cause an increased loss of calcium from the bones, which may cause osteoporosis leading to a gradual decrease in height.

303

REFERENCE

Nettina, S. M. (2007). *The Lippincott manual of nursing practice* (8th ed., Philippine ed.). Philadelphia: Lippincott Williams & Wilkins.

NCLEX-RN CATEGORY **Reduction of Risk Potential**

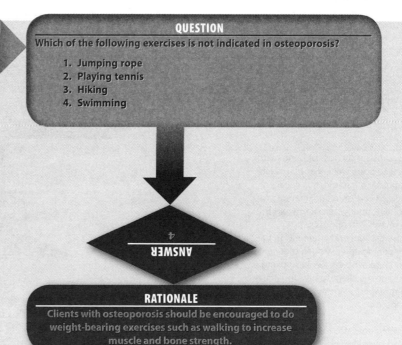

CONCEPT

Weight-bearing exercises are indicated to prevent osteoporosis.

QUESTION

Which of the following exercises is not indicated in osteoporosis?

1. Jumping rope
2. Playing tennis
3. Hiking
4. Swimming

POINTERS

- Osteoporosis is the loss of bone matrix leading to bone weakness making it susceptible to fracture. It is usually associated with smoking, menopause, immobility, and hyperparathyroidism.
- X-ray reveals osteoporosis.
- Increase calcium and vitamin D in the diet.
- Use of conjugated estrogen therapy for menopausal women. Avoid smoking.
- Encourage the client to perform active weight-bearing exercises like brisk walking, jumping rope, hiking, tennis, and ballroom dancing.
- Swimming does not meet the criteria for resistance needed to prevent osteoporosis.

ANSWER

4

RATIONALE

Clients with osteoporosis should be encouraged to do weight-bearing exercises such as walking to increase muscle and bone strength.

REFERENCE

Nettina, S. M. (2007). *The Lippincott manual of nursing practice* (8th ed., Philippine ed.). Philadelphia: Lippincott Williams & Wilkins.

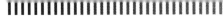

CONCEPT

Shortening and external rotation of the leg indicates a hip fracture.

POINTERS

- Hip fracture is a break in the continuity of the hip bone.
- Shortening and external rotation of the affected leg occurs.
- Diagnosed with X-ray
- Prepare the client for surgery.
- Postoperatively, maintain the legs in abduction by placing a wedge pillow between the legs.
- Monitor for signs and symptoms of complications (petechiae over the chest indicate fat embolism).

QUESTION

After a motor vehicle accident, which of the following clients needs to be assessed by the physician immediately?

1. A 35-year-old client with bruises on the arm
2. A 28-year-old with muscle cramps
3. A 30-year-old with shortening and external rotation of the right leg
4. A 29-year-old with hematoma on the thigh

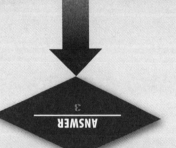

ANSWER

3

RATIONALE

Shortening and external rotation of the leg is indicative of a hip fracture.

REFERENCE

Nettina, S. M. (2007). *The Lippincott manual of nursing practice* (8th ed., Philippine ed.). Philadelphia: Lippincott Williams & Wilkins.

CONCEPT

Low impact exercises are allowed after hip surgery.

POINTERS

· Hip dislocation is manifested by:
  ▸ Shortened extremity
  ▸ Increased discomfort
  ▸ Inability to move the joints
· Home care considerations:
  ▸ Avoid excessive hip adduction, flexion, and rotation for 6 weeks after arthroplasty.
  ▸ Avoid sitting in a low chair.
  ▸ Avoid prolonged sitting (more than 30 minutes).
  ▸ Avoid activities that increase stress on the joint such as jogging, jumping, or lifting heavy loads.

QUESTION

Which of the following activities are allowed after hip replacement surgery? Select all that apply.

1. Walking
2. Playing golf
3. Dancing
4. Jogging
5. Jumping
6. Lifting heavy weights

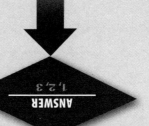

ANSWER

1, 2, 3

RATIONALE

A new hip is designed for low impact exercises such as walking, playing golf, and dancing. High impact exercises such as jogging may cause the prosthesis to loosen.

REFERENCE

Nettina, S. M. (2007). *The Lippincott manual of nursing practice* (8th ed., Philippine ed.). Philadelphia: Lippincott Williams & Wilkins.

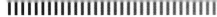

SUBJECT Fat Embolism Syndrome

CONCEPT

Respiratory distress and mental disturbances occur in fat embolism.

POINTERS

Risk factors for fat embolism
- Age (20–30, 60–70 years old)
- Multiple fractures of long bones

Early manifestations:
Confusion
Restlessness
Irritability
Disorientation

QUESTION

Which of the following manifestations are indicative of fat embolism? Select all that apply.

1. Crackles
2. Wheezes
3. Tachypnea
4. Restlessness
5. Fever
6. Petechiae in the mouth, chest, and axillary folds

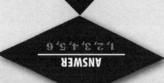

ANSWER 1, 2, 3, 4, 5, 6

RATIONALE

Crackles, wheezes, tachypnea, restlessness, fever, and petechiae in the mouth, chest, and axillary folds are all manifestations of fat embolism.

REFERENCE

Nettina, S. M. (2007). *The Lippincott manual of nursing practice* (8th ed., Philippine ed.). Philadelphia: Lippincott Williams & Wilkins.

SUBJECT Osteoarthritis

CONCEPT

Common risk factors for osteoarthritis are:
   Trauma
   Aging
   Obesity

POINTERS

- Osteoarthritis is a chronic, non-inflammatory degenerative joint disease.
- Degeneration of the articular cartilage in the joints occurs.
- Initially manifested by pain and swelling in a weight-bearing joint, usually aggravated by activity.
- The goal of care is to minimize discomfort.
- Implement:
   Weight control
   Hot compress or icepacks
   Aspirin use
   Trunk assistive devices (cane)

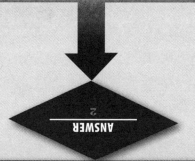

QUESTION

Which of the following questions should the nurse ask when assessing a client with osteoarthritis?

1. "Is your pain worse at night?"
2. "Did you have fractures before?"
3. "Don't you think your food has something to do with it?"
4. "Do you have joint stiffness in the evening?"

ANSWER
2

RATIONALE

Asking a client with osteoarthritis for any history of fractures in the past is assessing for a history of trauma, which is one of the contributing factors for osteoarthritis.

REFERENCE

Nettina, S. M. (2007). *The Lippincott manual of nursing practice* (8th ed., Philippine ed.). Philadelphia: Lippincott Williams & Wilkins.

CONCEPT

Visual hallucinations occur in delirium tremens.

POINTERS

- Delirium tremens usually occur 2–4 days after a client's last alcohol intake. Due to falling metabolism of alcohol, manifestations usually include coarse hand tremors, autonomic hyperactivity (high heart rate, high blood pressure, or sweating), seizures, anxiety, hallucinations (visual, tactile, or auditory), and insomnia.

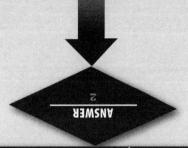

QUESTION

Which type of room is appropriate for a client with delirium tremens?

1. A darkened room
2. A well-lit room
3. A dimly lit room
4. A room with low-voltage incandescent bulbs

ANSWER

2

RATIONALE

It is important to provide the client a well-lit and quiet environment because clients with delirium tremens have hallucinations and they fear shadows.

309

REFERENCE

Gapuz, R. *The ABCs of passing foreign nursing exams.* Philippines: Gapuz Publications.

SUBJECT Methylergonovine Maleate (Methergine)

CONCEPT

Methergine initially causes hypertension.

QUESTION

Which of the following findings reflects a need to withhold methylergonovine maleate (Methergine)?

1. Respiratory rate of 14 per minute
2. Blood pressure of 160/110 mm Hg
3. Positive Brudzinski's sign
4. Negative Babinski reflex

POINTERS

- Methergine is an oxytocic; it is used as a treatment for postpartum atony and hemorrhage.
- Therapeutic effect is manifested as a firmly contracted uterus.
- Report difficulty of breathing.
- Monitor the BP because methergine causes hypertension.

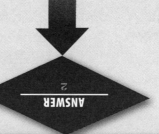

ANSWER

2

RATIONALE

Methergine should be withheld in a client with high blood pressure because it causes hypertension.

REFERENCE

Karch, A. M. (2007). *2008 Lippincott's nursing drug guide*. Philadelphia: Lippincott Williams & Wilkins.

CONCEPT

A client with acute physiologic alteration who is exhibiting symptoms of a complication is a priority.

POINTERS

- When answering questions related to prioritizing, focus on the following:
  ▸ Physiologic needs
  ▸ Acute conditions
  ▸ Signs of complications

QUESTION

Which of the following clients should the nurse attend to first?

1. A 3-year-old child with otitis media admitted for fever and earache
2. A 25-year-old manic client with hyperactivity and insomnia
3. A 30-year-old client with angina pectoris complaining of chest pain for the last 30 minutes
4. A 27-year-old gravida 2, para 1 client who is 8 months pregnant with a positive non-stress test

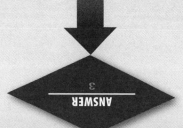

ANSWER

3

RATIONALE

The client with angina pectoris, who is complaining of chest pain for the last 30 minutes, has a physiologic problem that is acute.
Chest pain that is more than 20 minutes in duration is indicative of myocardial infarction, a possible complication of angina.

REFERENCE

Gapuz, R. *The ABCs of passing foreign nursing exams*. Philippines: Gapuz Publications.